In the Shadow

of

POLIO

In the Shadow

of

POLIO

A Personal and Social History

KATHRYN BLACK

⬩⬩

ADDISON-WESLEY PUBLISHING COMPANY

Reading, Massachusetts   Menlo Park, California   New York
Don Mills, Ontario   Harlow, England   Amsterdam   Bonn
Sydney   Singapore   Tokyo   Madrid   San Juan
Paris   Seoul   Milan   Mexico City   Taipei

Library of Congress Cataloging-in-Publication Data

Black, Kathryn.
    In the shadow of polio : a personal and social history / Kathryn
Black.
        p.   cm.
    Includes bibliographical references and index.
    ISBN 0-201-40739-6
    ISBN 0-201-15490-0 (pbk.)
    1. Black, Virginia, d. 1956—Health. 2. Poliomyelitis—Patients—
Arizona—Biography. I. Title.
RC181.U6A63 1996
362.1'96835'0092—dc20
[B]   95-43963
                                                                  CIP

Cover design by Suzanne Heiser
Text design by Barbara Cohen Aronica
Set in 11-point Bembo by Weimer Graphics, Indianapolis, IN
1 2 3 4 5 6 7 8 9-MA-0100999897
First printing, April 1996
First paperback printing, April 1997

To Virginia and Mary Ellen, still loved, still missed

We are healed of a suffering only by experiencing it to the full.

—Marcel Proust

CONTENTS

ACKNOWLEDGMENTS

This book contains many stories. It is first a story of my family, and I could not have told it without the memories of Del Black, my father; Ken Black, my brother; Maurine Royce, my grandmother; and Katherine Donald Geary, my cousin and godmother. I'm grateful to them for their willingness to talk to me of a painful time. I am also grateful to the "Polio Alums" in Seattle for their kindnesses to me and my mother, and for their memories. Most especially, I thank Marcelle Dunning, M.D., for opening her home to me, for sharing her unpublished papers, for providing medical detail, for reading the manuscript and offering helpful comments, and for encouraging me from the first telephone call.

This book also, however, includes the stories of many other people who lived with and remember polio. To the scores of people who allowed me to interview them and who wrote often long, detailed, and thoughtful letters to me, I am indebted. Hearing their stories not only strengthened my awareness of that time in history, but brought me comfort and courage as I struggled to tell what happened to my mother. Each letter and interview contributed something, historical fact or inspiration. A few of the people I encountered in my research are named in the book, and my debt to them is clear. To all the unnamed others, I offer my deepest thanks as well.

Thanks also to Carolyn Roberts for research assistance, to Krystyna Poray Goddu, Pamela Novotny, and Marian Faux for their friendship and insight, to Loretta Barrett, my agent, who stuck with me while I found the story I wanted to tell, and to Sharon Broll, my editor at Addison-Wesley, who really meant it when she said she was there for me.

Special thanks to Paula Bard, who was both safety net and cattle prod when the time finally came, almost a decade ago, for me to search for my past. She never let me down. Ditto for Laura Goodman, who is not only a dear friend but an extraordinary editor. She read every word of my manuscript, at least once, and asked hard questions, believing I could answer them.

Most of all, I thank Jens Husted and our sons, Ian and William, who keep me safe and loved. Together, we're creating new family memories.

P R O L O G U E

For most of my life, my father and I
have had separate homes in distant states. From the time I was six years
old, we had shared hardly more than a polite, once-a-year-Christmas-
card relationship, but I wasn't surprised when one day in late April
1988 he called me at my home in San Francisco. In the previous few
months we had warily begun to get reacquainted. I had visited him at
his home in Seattle, which marked the first time we'd been together in
almost ten years. I had gone because he had had surgery for a heart
aneurysm, and I was afraid he would die. His possible death didn't
dismay me for its potential loss in my life, because he had been lost to
me long ago. What I feared was that he might die before I found the
courage to ask him about the secrets in our family's history. He survived the surgery, and I cautiously began to pose questions.

After years of silence, we were talking on the telephone every
few weeks, though mostly about the present, his new relationship,
and my failing marriage. When he called that day in April, I expected
it to be another such conversation, but he surprised me by saying he
was feeling blue and had been thinking a lot about my mother. He
never spoke of her unless I asked, and although she was the secret I
most wanted revealed, in those days I seldom probed for information
about her. That morning, Dad told me he had been remembering
how our family used to camp out among the Joshua trees and saguaro
in the Arizona desert when we'd lived in Phoenix.

"Do you remember," he asked, "how your mother and I used
to fly kites with you and Kenny? How at night we would lie on cots
so the rattlers couldn't get us and listen to the coyotes?"

"No. I don't remember. I wish I did."

My father had once said that that first year in Arizona was the
happiest of his life, maybe the only happy time of his life. Maybe it

was my happiest time, too, and yet I couldn't conjure anything more than fleeting images that were like half-remembered dreams, heavy with emotion but divulging few details.

"These last few days," he continued, "I haven't been able to get those colorful kites off my mind. I don't know why."

In front of me was my desk calendar on which April 24 was circled in heavy, repeated pencil lines. I hesitated, then said, "Dad, do you know that yesterday was the anniversary of my mother's death?"

I HAD NO NAME FOR HER. When she was alive, I called her "Mommy." How could I call her that, now that I was thirty-eight and older than she'd ever become? "Mom" was too casual, too familiar. Her given name, Virginia, felt false. Speaking to my father of her, I could only say "my mother." She had been dead thirty-two years.

I LISTENED, WAITING FOR DAD'S RESPONSE. There was silence.

Then, a gurgled "No." He began to sob and choked out, "I have to hang up now."

The line clicked dead.

My fingers gripped the telephone receiver; my body tensed in a familiar effort to fight the rising emotion. Then I let it come. I hung up the telephone and put my head on my desk and wept.

Like my father, I'd worked hard for three decades to bury the memories of my mother's illness and death, but we had buried them alive. I had obscured my memories, shrouded them, ignored them, but all through the years they had pulsated with undiminished strength, never letting me wander far from the unacknowledged awareness of her absence.

Until I was in my late thirties, I had not known the date of my mother's death. I had been aware of it only in the same vague way as my father, as a troublesome tug from the subconscious, but I had never honored the day or known why the coming of spring would find me fighting depression instead of rejoicing in the new season. I knew nothing and had been told nothing about how and when she became ill. I had not even been aware that those were cavernous gaps in my history. When I look back on my ignorance, I'm amazed at how much I acquiesced in the don't-ask, don't-talk, don't-feel dictate of my family.

The few precious memories of the last two years of my mother's life that I carried through childhood and into adulthood swam like isolated, vibrant fish in an otherwise black sea. The part of ourselves that closes to protect us from what is too painful to remember darkened those final years of her life. I emerged after her death a second-grader with a past to hide, and to hide from.

That telephone call from my father in 1988 was the last in a series of events over the previous months that had told me I could no longer ignore my history. I was compelled to search for memory, for my own past. I wanted to know what had become of our family during the two years she lay paralyzed and helpless, breathing with a machine. I wanted to know about the disease that had killed my mother. And I wanted to find in the larger world what comfort I could in a connection with others who'd suffered from polio. I wanted to know whether the disease's impact on anyone else had been as profound as that on my family. Had that time truly disappeared without a sign, as it seemed to? Or did it still ring in the lives of others, as it did in mine? Slowly, as I learned my story and heard those of others, I began to fill in the dark holes, to give order, meaning, and rhythm to the pastiche of memory.

I FORCED MYSELF TO GIVE HER A NAME: *Mother.* I love the sound of it. I have never called anyone Mother. I like to think that if she were with me now I could say, "Mother," and she would look up and smile. Mother.

CHAPTER ONE

Backache

On a spring evening in 1954 my mother and I walked hand in hand to my brother's school, where a carnival was about to begin. These decades later I still see her in the lavender sundress that fit snugly over her hips, its wide straps reaching over her thin shoulders. She carried a matching jacket, cropped above the waist and short-sleeved, for the Arizona nights had been unusually chilly. I don't know where my brother, a first-grader, and my father were just then. Maybe they'd gone on ahead. This memory holds only four-year-old me and my smiling mother, her wispy light hair curled off her high forehead, her open-toed shoes clicking on the cement walk. I held on tightly.

We lived in a rented unit in a single-story housing complex near the center of Phoenix. The square, pastel stucco houses, each exactly like the next, angled around a grassy common area where a lone tree suggested shade and marked a gathering place for neighbors. We lived in number 483. The back door, the only one we used, opened into the one-room kitchen and living room; on the left were two small bedrooms and a bathroom. When the wind blew in the early spring, the scent from citrus orchards, just blocks away, sweetened our low-cost housing project, called Duppa Villa. Pick-your-own grapefruit and oranges were ours for pennies apiece.

The forties had brought a population boom to Phoenix with the addition of Luke and Williams Air Force Bases. Helping to ease the housing crisis and the plight of the city's needy citizens, the federal government funded projects like Duppa Villa, built on the poor side of the railroad tracks. They were spartan, but for those who in

4

the same location had been sheltered sometimes by nothing more than cardboard, the new developments meant a step up as America went to war.

By the time my family arrived, in 1953, the sameness of the complex had been mitigated by lawn and shrubbery and the lives of the hundreds of young families who lived there, and Phoenix boomed anew. The 1950 census put the population at just over 100,000, but in 1954 the city erected new signs at the edge of town announcing 140,062 residents.

Transplanted Coloradans, my parents, Virginia and Delbert Black, both aged twenty-eight, my brother, Kenny, and I learned desert ways in our new home. Every morning we checked for hiding scorpions before slipping our shoes on, and though we were forbidden to play barefoot, Kenny and I sometimes removed our shoes and pressed our feet against the cold, linoleum-covered cement floors. On weekends the four of us often set out for the desert with two or three canvas bags of water strapped to the car and camped in the land of rattlesnakes, coyotes, and javelinas. We explored dry creek beds, burned mesquite wood for campfires, flew kites, and swam in lakes. I know this because my father and brother remember and, when I asked, told me of the camping. At night, when we drove home, Ken tells me, the desert seemed to move as we traveled through it. It all, surely, was high adventure for a preschool girl, and I suppose those outings were what planted in me the seeds of my love of the desert Southwest, its serenity and hint of danger.

I do have one memory of my own from those outings. Daddy and I stood at the trunk of our Chevrolet. Kenny was in the distance, crouched, absorbed in something on the ground. I can't see Mother in this memory, she is behind us, but I feel her and know her to be there. I'm struck by how different that brief period of my life was when her presence, not her absence, was assumed. From the open trunk Daddy drew a bottle, poured himself a shot and swigged it, shivering and grimacing as it went down. "Why do you drink that if you don't like it?" I asked. He laughed and shook his head.

On weekdays, my father, in his cotton short-sleeved shirt and trousers went to a downtown job at a loan company, while Mother, like other mothers of the fifties, stayed at home, cooked big pots of spaghetti sauce, and did her ironing in front of television quiz shows.

I don't remember what I felt then, but I like to think I was contented, carefree, that we laughed a lot in our tiny apartment, that my parents loved each other and us. Now, however, all that I know about what was to come for our family colors those years with wistfulness and melancholy. It was the last time my mother and father and brother and I were together as an ordinary family. For that short time in the early fifties, we were normal—undistinguished by circumstances, expectations, or accomplishments.

THE KITCHEN TABLE, pushed up against the wall just inside the back door, anchored our home life. There Kenny and I ate watermelon and listened to *The Lone Ranger* and *Sky King* on a brown, round-shouldered radio. There, Mother sat to write letters home, to Colorado. After more than a year in Arizona she finally had the news she most wanted to send: our family was moving back. Throughout their marriage my parents had disagreed about their hometown. Mother wanted to live there, and Dad wanted to be anywhere else. Boulder was the site of painful, shameful growing-up memories for him, and by age twenty-eight my father had already settled on escape as the way out of life's troubles. But on May 31, 1954, Mother wrote a letter to her mother and father in Boulder saying that the company Dad worked for was transferring him to Denver. Mother had already persuaded him to return to Colorado without a transfer, so the news that the company would pay for our move and have a job waiting excited her. "Isn't that swell?" she wrote to her parents. We would be on our way before the end of June.

I have that letter and another sent just a few weeks before. Thirty years after they were mailed, I finally asked my grandmother for memories and mementos, and she gave them to me. My mother's letters reveal a family whose ups and downs seemed to rest on small details. A colorful "squaw" shirt from Dad and a handmade sun hat from Kenny for Mother's Day delighted her. An eleven-dollar doctor bill and fifty dollars laid out to the car mechanic in the same week caused her worry, but not enough to dampen her cheerfulness. She joked about the cookies she'd made for Kenny to take to school, saying one of his classmates had gone home sick; "but I really don't think they were that bad," she wrote to my grandmother.

When my grandmother received the letter saying our family now most certainly was returning to Colorado, she splurged on a long-distance call. She and Mother chatted and made plans for their reunion. Mother's exuberance over the move, and the pool party Dad's office mates were throwing for him, however, was dampened by a backache that had worsened over the past couple of days. She wasn't feeling well and hoped that whatever was ailing her would pass quickly. Mother would have to drive our Chevy sedan to Colorado while Dad drove the pickup. That long trip, she said to her mother, would be no fun with a bad back.

As my father remembers the story, the backache soon took a bad turn. He tried rubbing her muscles, and when that didn't help, he drove to a distant drugstore—the only one open on a Sunday evening—for aspirin and liniment, confident they would ease her discomfort. Groping for a simple, ordinary explanation for this intrusion, they told each other the packing must have strained her muscles.

I DON'T REMEMBER THE TELEPHONE CALL or the backache, but I do remember that each evening when I went to bed, a few feet from my sleeping brother in our shared bedroom, I'd lie there sucking my thumb in the not-yet dark, listening for the noises of insects and neighbors. Every night, I stayed awake until my father checked on Kenny and me. I always let my thumb droop loosely in my mouth, pretending to be asleep so that Daddy could pull it out, then place my hand on the pillow and softly close the door behind him. Keeping my eyes closed, enjoying the near-sleep, I'd find my thumb again. I wonder whether he came in that Sunday night or whether he was too preoccupied with my mother's backache to perform the ritual. I wonder whether I lay waiting, having to do without him and lull myself the whole way to sleep. I want—and can never have—every detail of those early days: the sound of my mother's voice, what she kept in her bureau drawers, what she and Dad talked about late at night, what the two of them hoped for in their lives and for their children. The weight of what I don't remember or never knew pulls me down, and only by trying to fill the holes in my not-knowing can I be released.

DESPITE THE DRUGSTORE AIDS, Mother passed the evening in increasing pain. Lifting her arms to put her hair in pincurls reminded her how stiff and achy her neck and shoulders were. Straightening up after bending over to pull off her shoes was difficult. Deep, cramping spasms ran up and down her legs and twitched in her back. As the night lengthened, the symptoms accumulated: pounding head pain, aching joints, shortness of breath, a strange sour taste, thirst. Her mind drifted and blanked, refusing her efforts to focus. She paced uncomfortably. After she finally dropped into bed, she noticed that she had trouble moving her legs when she rolled to her side. In the morning, Dad took her to a doctor. It was June 21.

Kenny went to school, and I was sent to stay with Tensia Garcia. She and her husband, Frank, a salesman for a beauty supply company, also lived in Duppa Villa and had become good friends to our family. We often exchanged dinner invitations, and Dad liked hearing Frank say that he knew no one else who could eat such hot food, especially a gringo. All these years later, I can remember aimlessly riding the rusted, hand-me-down tricycle that Kenny and I shared around the sidewalks of the communal square in the white, flat sunlight. I remember inspecting the faucet outside our apartment, a source of fearful fascination since the day Kenny had accidentally caught a scorpion in a mayonnaise jar held under the spigot. I remember idly watching a mother nurse her baby beneath the courtyard tree. I wonder now whether those memories are from that day with Mrs. Garcia, as I waited for my mother to come home.

THE DOCTOR EXAMINED MOTHER in his office and quickly made a diagnosis that startled my parents: polio. It had never occurred to them that *polio* could be the cause of her misery. Their experience with the disease was limited. They had had a high school classmate who, after graduation, had been paralyzed with polio, and our family had a five-thousand-dollar polio insurance policy through Dad's office, which they certainly hadn't expected to need. Almost daily the disease made the news, but never had they dreamed that polio would find our family.

The doctor was matter-of-fact and unalarmed as he ordered a spinal test for confirmation. Also called a lumbar puncture, the procedure required patients to curl into a fetal position to expose the spine to a needle through which fluid was drawn for analysis. If the patient had polio, the fluid showed cellular and chemical changes consistent enough for physicians to diagnose the disease. During epidemics, hospital emergency rooms were set up to do the taps to anyone coming in with fever or lassitude. The procedure was so common in one hospital that a jaded technician kept a book propped up to entertain himself while a patient's liquid dripped. For those whose spines were penetrated, however, the procedure was singular and not easily forgotten. Mother's puncture went smoothly, though not without discomfort.

Although the symptoms of headache, fever, malaise, upset stomach, and muscle pain were common to many viral infections, Mother's doctor probably suspected polio simply because the warm-weather polio season had begun. Arizona was not, however, having an epidemic, and 1954 was not expected to be a bad polio year for the state. When Mother fell ill, there were only twenty-eight other cases reported, compared to thirty-nine by the same date the year before. Many of those patients had been or were being cared for at Phoenix Memorial Hospital, one of the few hospitals in a wide area of the Southwest equipped to care for polio patients.

"Try not to worry," the doctor said, assuring Mother and Dad that she appeared to have a light case of nonparalytic polio, which, like most viruses, would run its course in a few days. "Expect full recovery," he told them. Yet despite his casual reassurance, the doctor immediately ordered Mother to Phoenix Memorial. No one knew how polio passed from person to person, but as it was clearly a contagious disease, health officials considered isolation of patients in the acute stages only prudent. Dad took Mother to the hospital, where a nurse led her to the polio ward.

Although forbidden to visit her, Dad walked around the sprawling wing of the one-story hospital until he found her window. He leaned in to talk and smuggle her a cigarette.

THE HOSPITAL HAD BEGUN as St. Monica's Mission, founded in 1934 by a Franciscan priest as a clinic for the poor. In 1942 it had outgrown its donated space in a former grocery store and had moved into a new structure built in a cotton field south of town. The war had made both funds and building materials scarce, resulting in a wood-frame and concrete-block building that seemed makeshift. "A flimsy shell" was how Dad saw it. Clearly, the developers had skimped on the architect, for the design, compartmentalized rather than integrated, was as simple as if imagined by a young child. A flat, rectangular building at one end housed the entrance, reception area, and administrative offices. From it stretched a long, wide hallway with five flat, rectangular wings jutting to each side.

The nonprofit, private St. Monica's has been sold to the federal government in 1947, and in 1949 it had been renamed Memorial Hospital to honor the war dead. In 1951, because of the growing legions of polio victims, a wing once set aside solely for pediatrics had been converted to a polio ward for both children and adults. What the hospital lacked in physical amenities, it made up for in services. By 1954, when Mother lay in the polio ward, the hospital staff had had ample experience caring for polio victims. At times, up to seventy iron lungs packed patient rooms, a solarium, and the hallway. On staff were nurses and doctors with special training in the care of polio patients. Their wing was equipped with a rocking-bed ward, an iron-lung ward, and a physical therapy room. The day Mother arrived, nurses applied moist hot packs to her back and legs, bringing relief from the pain and spasms. A board placed under the mattress gave additional comfort to her back.

DAD FINALLY WAVED GOODBYE TO HER from the window and went home to call her parents, Maurine and Hayes Royce, with the news. Even though he tried to reassure them, repeating what the doctor had said about it being a mild case, they were horrified by the possibilities that hung on the word *polio*. In 1954, few people could hear the diagnosis and not be dismayed. A decade of polio summers, the high-profile March of Dimes fund-raising, and word of a vaccine's development had kept the disease in the news. Almost everyone knew someone who had been touched by polio—a friend, a neighbor, a colleague. Still, most people, like my grandparents and parents, knew only that the disease could cripple. What this diagnosis of polio meant, what Mother's outlook might be, and how long it would be before anyone could say for sure were all mysteries to my family.

The telephone conversation between Dad and my grandparents must have been stilted. Theirs had always been an uneasy alliance, something I'd grown up feeling and seeing, and this surely was difficult news to deliver about their only child. Maurine and Hayes had disapproved of Dad since my parents' high school days together. Dad remembers, "Maurine was never nice, and Hayes didn't talk to me." One time, Delbert had come to the door to pick up Virginia for a date, and Maurine had sent him away, saying her daughter wasn't there; in fact, Virginia had been inside waiting and wondering why her date had stood her up.

MY GRANDPARENTS LIVED near the University of Colorado, next door to the house where my grandfather had grown up. He and Maurine built a one-bedroom red brick bungalow in the yard where Hayes had kept mules as a boy. When Virginia was born, they added a room.

Mother's friends were the children of professionals and university people, though my grandfather was a postman, not a professor. Throughout the Great Depression, Hayes, like most other postal workers, stayed employed, a fact that considerably enhanced the family's blue-collar existence. Despite the poverty around them, they never missed a meal or stood in line for food and could even afford to go to a picture show now and then. Nonetheless, as with so many others of those depression-era generations, those years instilled in my grandparents a persistent sense of the wolf at the door.

As my grandmother tells it, my mother was a model child who earned good grades, wanted to be a nurse, and played the oboe in the high school orchestra. I borrowed yearbooks from one of her classmates and learned that she was in the French Club and was vice-president of the band. Candid photos showed her sitting on a rock with several friends in the mountains near Boulder and drinking from a soda bottle. When she was a junior, the graduating seniors wrote up a mock will, turning over their high school pleasures and possessions to the upcoming seniors. Virginia and three of her best friends were willed a booth at the Tiptop Cafe, the local hangout. One of her classmates told me that her two best friends, who could have told me the most, both died young.

With blond hair swept high off his forehead, Delbert was the handsome rebel-without-a-cause. A promising sprinter on the track team as a sophomore, he had a burst of growth that added nearly a foot to his height, aborting his glory and taking away his speed—but not, apparently, his charm. The youngest of seven children, he had an appealing vulnerability that was not a device to attract attention but a real sense, acquired at his father's deathbed years before. His father, Jesse Black, had died of gallstones at age forty-five; he had refused the operation that could have saved him, apparently preferring a painful death to a surgeon's knife. When Jesse died, Delbert was four years old and his eldest sister was twenty-one. His mother, Maud, began cooking at a cafeteria and then for fraternities to keep her family going. Dad grew up poor, defending himself against loneliness, rejection, and his three older brothers.

Delbert and Virginia graduated from Boulder High School in 1942 in the wake of Japan's attack on Pearl Harbor. Dad enlisted in the U.S. Marine Corps and, after completing boot camp, put in a request to join the Raiders, a battalion modeled after British commandos specializing in clandestine strikes. As Delbert saw it, they went on suicide missions, which was just the kind of action he wanted. His drill instructor, however, refused to grant the assignment and told Delbert, "You'll thank me for this in twenty-five years." The marines took him to Saipan, Iwo Jima, and Okinawa, where in an air detachment he flew in B-25s attacking enemy ships by night. The war ended with him in Okinawa, as a master sergeant. Although he remembers his military years fondly, as a time when he felt successful, he apparently never considered staying in the service and took his discharge. With no plans for his future, he went home to Colorado.

After graduating from high school, Virginia enrolled at the University of Colorado and then transferred to St. Anthony's Hospital in Denver, where she was a cadet nurse. There, much to my grandmother's delight, she became engaged to a young obstetrician. Soon after accepting his ring, she assisted him at a birth and announced to her cousin, Katherine Donald, "We had our first baby together yesterday." But try as she might, she couldn't make the future promised by that young man suit her, nor could she get Delbert off her mind. Although they had dated but a few times, and she had written to him only occasionally during the war, she decided she didn't want the young doctor or nursing school—she wanted Delbert. When he showed up in Denver, tanned and fit, in the fall of 1945, she told him she had made up her mind to quit school and give back the ring. A year later, on September 3, 1946, they eloped.

Recently I found a snapshot taken on their wedding day. I keep it framed in my office and look at it often, wishing I could time-travel and talk to those two young people who, because of what I don't know about them and should know, seem more like strangers than strangers. She was twenty, and he had just turned twenty-one. In the photo they stand pressed together, heads tilted toward one another, my mother gripping one of Dad's hands in both of hers. She's looking at him with half-closed eyes and a stifled smile; clearly, she adores him. His body and amused gaze point at the camera, and he holds a cigarette in his free hand. He looks caught, and pleased.

WHEN SHE HEARD THE NEWS over the telephone that Virginia was in the hospital with a case of polio, my grandmother could not be reassured. Nor would she sit home waiting for further word; she and Hayes packed the car and started the eight-hundred-mile drive to Phoenix the next day. They were already on the road when early the following morning Dad answered a knock at the door and was startled to see a police officer standing on our step. "Mr. Black?" he said. "You're needed at the hospital."

Mother was worse. Much worse. Her case was *not* mild. She had bulbospinal polio, a combination of two types of paralytic polio, spinal and bulbar. This was the most dire of diagnoses.

MY GRANDPARENTS ARRIVED THE NEXT DAY and learned the bad news: Mother was gravely ill. They went straight to the hospital. Maurine still balks at talking of that day, and I can only imagine the fear she and Hayes must have suffered when they were told to put on white sterile gowns and masks and were led down a corridor smelling of disinfectant and littered with metal medicine carts and wheel-chairs. A nurse guided them past rooms of polio patients to an iron lung. Wards of tank respirators looked something like the boiler rooms of giant ships, with the blur of gauges, tubes, latches, and dials. The six-foot metal cylinders that breathed for patients lay like coffins on stands that raised them to table height. Intravenous bottles hung from aluminum poles next to respirators, and at one end of each lay a head. Rectangular windows, through which parts of bodies could be glimpsed, and a row of three or four portholes, used by nurses to tend to the bodies inside, lined the sides of the iron lungs.

A respirator's rhythmic *ka-thum-pa* sounds and the cacophony of mechanized, wheezing breath led them to Mother. The iron lung encased Virginia in a vacuum. Pumps working at regular intervals applied first positive, then negative pressure, pushing on her lungs to expel air, then pulling on them to draw more in—an awkwardly con-sistent cadence. In this acute, dangerous stage of the disease, Mother likely lay semiconscious, unable to speak. One tube entered her nose, and another penetrated her neck.

At the sight of her daughter's gaunt face protruding from the massive iron cylinder, my grandmother gasped, then paled as she reeled with dizziness. A nurse took her arm and led her to a chair, command-ing her to lower her head. The hospital allowed only short visits to patients still in the acute stages of polio, and time was almost up when my grandmother felt steady enough to cross the room to Mother.

My grandmother had brought along a gift for that first hospital visit: a white quilted bathrobe with white velvet ribbons. When she told me that detail, I wept, imagining my grandmother selecting that pristine and utterly inappropriate gift for the daughter who, any day up to that one, would have loved its elegance and beauty. The robe would have been jarringly out of place amid the metal and glass and rubber tubing, where the space between life and death pressed to a thin line. How little my grandmother knew—how little most people knew—of the grim particulars of this disease. The last time she'd seen her, Mother had been a healthy, active woman, concerned that she didn't have a new bathing suit for the upcoming office pool party and pleased that her son had joined the best readers in his class.

Polio had not left Mother lying prettily against fluffed white pillows but palsied, in a torpor. A rubber collar separated her head from her body, her brown hair was matted from perspiration and fell back from her face, and her long, slender neck was marred by a raw, sunken hole and a metal fixture holding a rubber tube. During her first night in the hospital, when the virus had raged through her body, deadening muscle after muscle but leaving her on fire with pain, doctors had performed an emergency tracheotomy to keep her from suffocating. The incision, a slice in the throat just below the Adam's apple, made a hole in the windpipe where an oxygen tube could be inserted and from which phlegm could be drawn, saving her from drowning on the mucus that obstructed her upper respiratory passages. Her throat muscles useless, she was unable to breathe, cough, or swallow on her own. The tracheotomy signaled to all at the hospital that Mother was among the sickest, highest-risk polio patients.

SPINAL POLIO, IN WHICH THE VIRUS ATTACKS the motor nerve cells of the spinal cord, causes damage ranging from weakness in one muscle to complete quadriplegia. It is the least likely type of polio to kill its victims, unless, as in my mother's case, it attacks the respiratory muscles, and then up to 50 percent of victims die. The poliovirus, which can invade any of the motor cells of the spinal cord and brain stem, has, like many other viruses, an unexplained specific appetite. It leaves unscathed the dorsal sensory cells, which receive incoming messages such as pain, temperature, position, balance, and vibration, preferring the nearby anterior horn cells, which send messages of movement to the skeletal muscles of the body—arms, legs, abdomen, chest, and neck. This means that if a hand paralyzed by polio were placed on a hot stove burner, it would feel the heat through the healthy dorsal cells. But no matter how urgent the messages the brain sent to remove that hand, it would stay, flesh burning, the destroyed anterior cells unable to do their job of relaying the signals to the hand.

In spinal polio, any combination of anterior horn cells can be affected, but legs are more often involved than arms, and the large muscle groups of the hands more often than the small ones. Any combination of limbs might be paralyzed, though most commonly it is one leg, followed by one arm, or both legs and both arms. Paralysis sometimes occurs within a few hours, but it often spreads over two or three days and ends with the breaking of the fever. During the first night Mother was in the hospital, the virus had swept through her body, disengaging muscle after muscle, including her intercostals and diaphragm.

All that would have been bad enough, but the virus worked at the bulbar cells of her central nervous system also, causing severe respiratory difficulties by another route. When the poliovirus heads for the brain, it can attack cranial nerves that control eye and facial muscles and interfere with chewing, which causes victims considerable difficulty but is not life-threatening. More commonly, however, bulbar polio attacks cranial nerves that operate the pharynx, the soft palate, and the larynx, making swallowing, breathing, and speaking difficult or impossible, and endangering the life of victims.

At the initial onslaught, Mother struggled to maintain even slow, irregular, shallow breaths. The doctors and nurses at Phoenix Memorial stood by, knowing that at any moment she could die. No case of polio was considered routine, but respiratory cases caused considerable turmoil. As paralysis overtook Mother, aides lifted her onto the bed of an iron lung, on hand for just such an emergency. They carefully straightened her body and rolled the cotlike slab into its cylindrical tank, clamping it shut tightly. The rubber collar around her neck prevented air from escaping, and cotton padding reduced chaffing as the rubber slid up and down her neck with each breath. Her shoulders wedged against one end of the tank, her feet set firmly against a foot board at the other, she lay entombed, but alive.

How to help victims suffering bulbospinal polio sometimes posed dilemmas for physicians, because treatments for the two kinds of paralysis conflicted. Doctors had to make difficult decisions about whether to perform tracheotomies, in particular. Tracheotomies had been discovered in the early forties and could save the lives of patients at risk of drowning in their own saliva. (Under normal circumstances a person secretes about a quart every twenty-four hours, and the amount can be much more with a disease of the nervous system like polio.) But because tracheotomies brought their own complications—such as infection, bleeding, and mucous plugs in the trachea, along with much distress to the patient—physicians often tried to delay or avoid them. With bulbar polio the operation could be avoided, if skillful caregivers helped the patient get rid of the saliva, and if the patient didn't panic. In this way physicians hoped to ease bulbar patients through the pharyngeal paralysis, which they knew might last only a few days, without opening the throat.

Iron lungs also posed risks for bulbar patients, who sometimes died in the tanks as they lay flat on their backs and aspirated their own secretions. Others died of exhaustion, fighting the machine that did not synchronize with the efforts of their unaffected breathing muscles.

In my mother's case, however, the virus so ravaged her body with both spinal and bulbar paralysis that her physicians had no qualms about placing her in an iron lung and doing a tracheotomy. Her rapid pulse, high blood pressure, irregular breathing, and bluish discoloration of the skin all called for life-saving measures. The tracheotomy and the tank respirator saved her that first night, but no one caring for her had confidence she would survive, nor could they predict what her condition would be if she did.

Mother hovered near death for days, her temperature and blood pressure dangerously high. She received around-the-clock care, but no medication could check the progress of the poliovirus, and no doctor dared give a barely breathing patient a sedative or painkiller. All her attendants could do was suction her fluids, monitor her breathing, and wait for the crisis to pass. The overall mortality rate for polio victims was less than one in ten, but 60 percent of those stricken with bulbospinal died. Twenty-five percent of polio deaths came in the first twenty-four hours, and Mother had passed that marker. But another lay ahead: 85 percent of deaths occurred during a victim's first twenty days in the hospital. Mother lay through those three weeks, in her tank, eyes closed, saliva from her parted lips carving a pink, raw line across her face, inhaling, exhaling, inhaling, exhaling.

She survived night after night. And the fever retreated. With the initial crisis past, she regained consciousness, but given her circumstance, which took her far from all familiar landmarks in her life, her awareness was limited. She couldn't move a muscle below her neck. Watery noises escaped through her tracheotomy tube; her tank pumped and whooshed. My grandparents and father continued their vigil through long, uneventful days. "The nightmare commenced," Dad recalled. "We watched her go from a healthy girl to a skeleton who couldn't breathe, strangling on her own saliva."

Time lost its familiar context, and uncertainty and foreboding colored those who kept vigil. Doctors had no news. My grandparents and father entreated the doctors to tell them how she fared. How long would she be in the hospital? What would happen to her?

"She's doing as well as can be expected," came the answer. "Only time will tell."

The unspoken and unquestioned implication was that "time" meant "a long time."

I DON'T KNOW WHERE my brother and I were during those days. My grandmother and father don't remember, and I have no memory of my mother's hospitalization in Phoenix. Perhaps we were with the Garcias or with the mother of one of Dad's friends from work, Mrs. Woodruff, who had taken care of us one day when Mother and Dad had gone to Mexico. All I know for certain is that wherever it was, I was waiting anxiously for Mother to come home, for Daddy to pull my thumb from my mouth and tuck me in, for my grandparents to give me piggyback rides and read to me. When I finally pieced together the story, I saw where my lifelong habit of waiting, with time as the enemy and vigilance my duty, had begun.

CHAPTER TWO

Epidemic of Fear

Growing up without my mother, I often searched for surrogates, and Martha Hoover, one of my favorites, lasted through many years. The single mother of my schoolmate Leona, she worked as a nurse to support her own mother and three children. She was accepting and kind, and best of all, seemed interested in me.

The Hoover family, like mine, had a past darkened with polio. Leona's younger sister, Penny, walked with a limp on a leg withered in the characteristic way of polio. And I knew that Leona's father, Ted, had died young, but I was unsure about the cause of death. None of us talked of the past—not Martha, not Leona, certainly not me. The memories were too painful to revisit, but I suspect that similar sorrows bound us unconsciously. When I finally approached Martha thirty-five years after polio had found her family, I heard in detail a story of how capricious and virulent the disease can be. And how even in 1953, the year following the worst polio epidemic in history, the disease was still misdiagnosed and denied.

Trouble for the Hoovers started on a hot, late August Sunday in 1953. Ted awakened with a pressure-cooker headache, and all three of the children—Leona, age four; Steve, three; and Penny, two—appeared to be coming down with something. Leona complained that her head hurt, but the others were too young to say what their trouble was. All were cranky and listless.

Martha was concerned about the children, but thought that Ted, thirty-three and as athletic as he had been when they met in 1945, was suffering from overwork and tension. They were getting ready to move from Miltonvale, Kansas, to Downs, sixty miles west on Highway 24. Ted had just finished six years of teaching history and coaching track, football, and basketball at Miltonvale High, and he had landed a new job at a bigger school. Monday morning, he rose early, packed the car, and headed to Downs to begin a week of teachers' meetings and to get his new football team ready for the season.

Alone with the children, Martha, a trained nurse, monitored their illnesses. She wondered whether they might have eaten too much fruit; they had all been feasting on peaches from the tree behind the farmhouse where they lived. Even in the early morning, the Kansas heat choked the small rooms, and she lay her three ailing children on a blanket on the living-room floor in front of a fan. The temperature and drought that summer were as severe as the country had seen since the mid-1930s. Erratic hot winds kept the air thick with dust, and the fan gave small comfort to the feverish, aching children.

As the days passed, Martha became more worried. Three times during the week, she borrowed a car from her landlord and friend, Lena, and took the children to three different doctors. Each told Martha to take them home. "It's the flu," they said. Still, polio hovered in the back of her mind. Martha asked each doctor, "What about polio? Couldn't it be polio?" Each doctor reassured her that it was not. No, they said, this isn't polio. The cold symptoms, the stomach upset, the fevers all pointed to flu.

Toward the end of the week, Leona and Steve got up from the blanket and began to play again, but two-year-old Penny, whimpering and frail, continued to lie hour after hour. Then, on Friday afternoon, Ted pulled up in his car, but it wasn't the homecoming Martha had been looking forward to. He was too sick to climb the stairs alone. Martha put him in a tub of hot water, and bathed his head and shoulders with a cloth. He begged for a painkiller, and Martha drove twenty miles to the nearest doctor to get a prescription for codeine. The drug helped Ted through the night, but on Saturday morning he couldn't stand up. With the help of a friend, Martha drove him to the hospital in Salina.

Doctors immediately diagnosed bulbar poliomyelitis. When Martha heard that, she ran down the hospital hallway in search of a telephone. She called Lena. "Get Penny here. *Now*. It's polio. I know she has it, too. Get her here as fast as you can."

When Lena arrived with Penny, a nurse called Martha to see her. By that time Penny's back was clenched in a stiff arch. Martha stayed only a few moments. She could not watch as the nurses applied moist, scorching wool packs to her daughter's tiny body. Penny's cries pierced the ward as doctors tried to loosen her muscles.

The hospital was short on nurses. When afternoon came, a doctor asked Martha if she would take the night shift and care for Ted herself. Of course, she said, and the nurse who had been with him left. Martha was alone with her husband as his paralysis spread, and as he lost the ability to swallow. He gasped each irregular breath. Martha suctioned the pooling fluids from his throat and talked softly to him, trying to calm the panic that made his breathing even more difficult. He choked again and again. He looked at her. "Save me," he whispered. "I'm a nurse," Martha thought. "Why *can't* I save him?"

Through the night she shared his every shallow, desperate breath, and then, just before dawn on Sunday, August 23, 1953, Ted died. Penny lay in another hospital bed suffering the acute, painful stages of the disease. She survived with muscles in her abdomen, back, right shoulder, and right leg paralyzed.

MARTHA HOOVER NEVER REMARRIED. For her, like many survivors, the second-guessing has never stopped. She still regrets having nursed Ted herself, believing she should have been able to save him or that some other nurse or doctor could have. She's still plagued by what-ifs: What if Ted had rested for a week instead of going to the new school? Did exertion in the early stages make his case fatal? What if she had taken Penny to the hospital earlier? Could the outcome have been different for all her family?

I've learned, talking with Martha and dozens of other polio families and victims, that most of us have unanswered and unanswerable questions about polio. For myself, I've resisted, but can't help asking, the truly futile one that rises so easily in the wake of disaster: *Why?* Why was *my* mother one to suffer this cruel disease? The answers I want, and expect comfort from, fall in the spiritual realm. The answers I've found are more pedestrian, but bring some comfort as well. My mother got polio simply because she was unlucky enough to have lived for twenty-eight years before encountering the poliovirus. Oddly, modern sanitation, which helped stem other infectious diseases such as tuberculosis, cholera, and typhoid, put her and whole populations of her peers and their children at risk.

Until the twentieth century the poliovirus was probably endemic, an unnoticed part of everyday life, silently infecting infants through fecal contamination of water and food. For centuries no one associated the disease's vague and inconsistent early symptoms—fever, headache, nausea, sore throat, stiffness—with the occasional, surprising paralysis, or even death, of a child. Where those crippling deformities came from mystified generation after generation of parents and doctors. Unknown to them, poliomyelitis spread from one susceptible child to another, creating a natural, almost universal immunity through mainly harmless and inapparent infections occurring at very early ages. For centuries, other childhood afflictions—smallpox, plague, distemper, and diarrheal disease—contributed to a high infant mortality rate and overshadowed polio.

Even though polio remains the only common disease that can cause sudden paralysis in otherwise healthy children, attempts to trace its origins have failed. Many accounts of lameness or withered limbs in children date back to Homer and the Bible, but the descriptions are too vague to pin them to polio. Archeological evidence, however, reveals that polio has been with us since at least 1500 B.C. An Egyptian stele from that period depicts a priest leaning on a staff, one leg withered and shortened with the foot dropped in a way characteristic of paralytic polio. In 1911 a Danish physician made a retro-diagnosis of the ancient priest's malady that has remained unchallenged.

Not until the end of the eighteenth century, however, did scientists first identify and describe the disease, and not until 1887 was the first epidemic noted, in Stockholm. The 44 cases reported there by pediatrician Karl Oscar Medin marked the beginning of epidemic waves of polio that would roll across much of the world, especially Europe, North America, and developed areas of the Southern

Hemisphere. The first U.S. outbreak, in Rutland, Vermont, struck 132 people in 1894. Just twenty-two years later, in 1916, the disease hit 29,000 people in the United States, killing 6,000, a number that remained a benchmark for decades.

IN THE TWENTIES POLIO WAS DEEPLY FEARED, but it was accepted as an unfortunate fact of life until it struck one particular man, radically altering its path in history. In August 1921, at the age of thirty-nine, Franklin Delano Roosevelt, the vigorous and prominent former assistant secretary of the navy under President Woodrow Wilson contracted a severe case of paralytic polio. Unwilling to accept his crippled state, FDR tried for years to walk on his useless legs. One summer, while visiting a friend's place at Horseneck Beach in Massachusetts, Roosevelt crawled with his arms in the hot sand dunes in hopes that the searing heat would strengthen his legs. In 1924 a friend told him that another polio victim had received helpful therapy from warm mineral water in the South. Roosevelt promptly visited the rundown resort in Warm Springs, Georgia, and the buoyant waters brought comfort and strength, if not regeneration, to his withered limbs. Other polio victims followed, and soon the president-to-be was teaching the newcomers his exercises and answering to "Dr. Roosevelt."

Some of the paying guests, however, objected to being around the twisted bodies and refused to eat in the same dining room. Money solved that problem, as it was to solve many others to come in the crusade against polio. In 1926, Roosevelt bought the entire property—twelve hundred acres in all, including the inn, cottages, springs, and pools—for $195,000 and invited people immobilized from polio to use the facilities. His law partner, Basil O'Connor, drew up papers to incorporate the nonprofit Warm Springs Foundation, and so, without any particular plan in mind, began the country's first organized effort to do something about polio.

Over the years, FDR and others continued to use Warm Springs for therapy and rehabilitation, but by the time he was elected president in 1933 and the Great Depression had settled on the country, the resort was broke. In a meeting of the spa trustees, someone proposed the idea of fund-raising by celebrating the president's birthday with balls all around the country. On the evening of January 30, 1934, people gathered in New York, Chicago, Newark, Palm Beach, Cleveland, Pittsburgh, Philadelphia, and Washington, D.C., to dance to "Did You Ever See a Dream Walking?" and other popular tunes of the time. Roosevelt, who turned fifty-two that day, announced to the nation: "This is the happiest birthday I have ever known." "The President's Birthday Ball Commission for Infantile Paralysis Research" was born, and the balls became an annual event, spreading to more and more cities and hotels, and the money poured in. Before long, however, the commission, which had been closely associated with the popular, but increasingly controversial president, was disbanded, and the National Foundation for Infantile Paralysis (NFIP) was established. With fanfare, the president pledged in 1938 that the new organization would make "every effort to ensure that every responsible research agency in this country [would be] adequately financed to carry on investigation into the cause of infantile paralysis and the methods by which it [might] be prevented."

Organizers soon hit on the idea of broadening the January take by asking people to send money directly to the White House. The singer Eddie Cantor, attending a meeting in Los Angeles on the MGM movie lot, suggested that stars take to the radio and ask people to send their dimes directly to the president at the White House. "We could call it the 'March of Dimes'!" he said, in a burst of marketing genius. The radio pleas worked. The first day, 30,000 letters landed in the White House mail room, compared to 5,000 on a normal day. Fifty thousand arrived the second day; 150,000, the third. With the White House mail room swamped in mail bags, no one could find the official mail. Dimes came baked into cakes, jammed into cans, glued to pictures of the president, and jingling loose in envelopes. In all, $268,000—2,680,000 dimes—came in for that first March of Dimes.

The NFIP fell into place just in time. Important questions about the disease needed to be answered by research: Did one or several polio viruses exist? How did polio enter into, travel through, and leave the body? Could vaccines be made that would prevent the disease?

Answers to these questions were imperative as the years 1939 through 1941 saw a record total of new cases—almost twenty-seven thousand—in the United States. In January 1942, the physician John C. Curran of the NFIP warned that this new high incidence was of "alarming significance" because it indicated that the disease was "getting a foothold in America." He was right. In 1941, New York State alone saw a 400 percent rise in cases over the previous year's number. By 1946 the worst epidemic of poliomyelitis since the 1916 outbreak gripped the United States. In one week in August 1946, twelve hundred cases were reported.

The disease crept into Tom Green County, Texas, in early June 1949 and found two preschool boys in the Fuentes family and three children in the Martin family. The virus spread, and soon, in a scene repeated in communities countrywide throughout the forties and fifties, anxious parents began carrying their feverish, aching children to doctors and hospitals. Tom Green's schools and swimming pools, along with the DeLuxe Bowling Alley and the San Angelo Roller Rink, closed. And still, by midsummer more than two hundred children and adults there had been swept up in polio's wake.

WHAT CAUSED THIS SHIFT from endemic to epidemic? Nothing more dramatic than a cleaner environment. Viruses, particles of genetic material that can invade human cells and cause ailments as benign as common warts or as devastating as AIDS, need a population of susceptible people in order to survive. For centuries, infants provided the poliovirus a steady supply of hosts, and open sewers delivered the disease to them. But as modern hygienic practices developed, increasing numbers of people escaped babyhood and even childhood without coming into contact with the virus.

Rather than being a disease of filth and poverty, as so many other serious contagious maladies are, polio acts in the opposite way, flourishing in highly developed countries. As countries such as the United States and Sweden raised their standards of living, they began to experience polio epidemics of greater size and severity because their populations hadn't gained immunity through exposure, while poor countries, with their crowding and primitive sanitation, continued to hardly notice the disease.

Epidemic somewhere in the United States almost every year from 1900 until 1956, polio slowly came to be seen as a common contagion affecting not only infants but also children and teenagers and, occasionally, young adults. When polio emerged as a disease of older children, it threatened entire generations in terrifying, mysterious epidemics that grabbed public attention. Generally a mild or even invisible infection in the young, the disease mysteriously often cripples or kills older victims. The Swedish epidemic of 1908 through 1911 established that mortality was lowest in children under five and rose with age.

Before the twentieth century it was virtually unheard of that a twenty-eight-year-old woman, like my mother, would get polio, but as the epidemics advanced, the age of onset increased. In 1916, 95 percent of the cases occurred in children under nine years old. By 1955, 25 percent of the victims were over age twenty. Individual communities saw their own sharp increases in adult cases, with devastating results. In 1953 in King County, Washington, for example, which includes Seattle, 41 percent of the victims were over age twenty-one.

In the forties researchers knew that the average age of children afflicted by polio was slightly lower in large cities than in country districts, which told them that merely growing older did not protect one from polio. They concluded that the relative immunity of adults was acquired through actual contact with the disease, since opportunity for contact comes earlier in crowded cities than in rural areas. This also gave them another important clue in understanding this mysterious disease: Apparently, the majority of people gained their immunity by having had the disease without ever knowing it. One woman told me that in 1946 her baby girl, a precocious, energetic child, fell ill but recovered in a few days. Afterward the girl's physical development slowed, and after a few months her mother took the girl to a specialist, who examined the child and said: "Only the good Lord can really tell you, but from everything we have found, evidently she had polio." He advised the parents to buy the girl a large, heavy tricycle, which she rode all through the house, reaching the pedals with the help of wooden blocks, to strengthen her legs. The remedy was effective.

With the epidemics came greater knowledge and a different attitude toward the disease, reflected in the change in its name. By the 1940s not only was the disease no longer confined to children, but it was far more widespread than reflected in the victims who became paralyzed. The term *infantile paralysis* was outdated, giving way by 1947 to the more scientific, formal name of *poliomyelitis*, meaning inflammation (*itis*) of the spinal cord (*myelos*) gray anterior matter (*polios*). Before long, the disease was neither formal nor distant, and, to fit headlines and daily conversation, it became simply *polio*.

THE DISEASE CAME INTO ITS STRENGTH in the United States from 1942 through 1953, with epidemics of unprecedented size, peaking in the summer of 1952 with almost sixty thousand cases. The virus leap-frogged across the country unpredictably. In 1944 and 1945 the Atlantic Seaboard was the center of outbreaks. In 1946 the Midwest, from the Appalachians to the Rockies, was hit hardest. Minneapolis, home to the world-famous Elizabeth Kenny Institute for the treatment of polio, took the sad distinction of having the worst polio outbreak of any U.S. city. By mid-August that year, 445 city residents had polio, 28 had died of the disease, and the city took on 300 other polio patients who were transferred in from around the state for care. In a single week in 1946, polio played no favorites; it struck a six-week-old baby in Chicago and a sixty-two-year-old farmer in Kansas. One of the Minneapolis victims was the three-year-old daughter of the physician John F. Pohl, a medical supervisor at the Kenny Institute. It was an unnecessary reminder that no person and no place was out of reach of the poliovirus. Between 1948 and 1955 there were more polio cases than in the previous thirty years.

In the summer of 1955 an epidemic hit Massachusetts, resulting in almost four thousand cases, the majority of which were paralytic, many of them adult bulbar cases requiring iron lungs. Boston's hospitals—not only those for contagious disease but also nearly all others—swelled with polio patients. At Massachusetts General, William Tisdale was a second-year medical resident in the emergency room. The summer was hot and tempers short, he remembered, and the twelve-hour work shifts seemed endless. "We were running scared," he recalled. "We were exhausted, depressed by what we'd seen." Another doctor there that summer told me that he had to "steel" himself to the task of coping "with what was a desperate situation." One "devastating night," the physician remembered, several patients in the respiratory ward died. "We tried to look at what we had done and whether we could have done any better," he said. They tried to find comfort in knowing they had done their best.

Thomas Whitfield was the pediatric assistant resident that summer at Massachusetts General. What stands out in his memory of the time is "a feeling of ominous foreboding and fear that started towards the end of June, maybe mid-June." The cases started early and kept going, with new patients arriving daily. The overworked doctors learned to stop for a few minutes and nap, heads down on desks or tables. In their few hours off, they went home to their wives and children and wondered whether they had brought polio with them. "We were frightened all the time," Whitfield remembered of that summer. Not only did doctors not know what to expect from the illness, which could be mild or fatal, but, of course, they feared getting it themselves. They washed their hands a lot, but they knew that didn't keep physicians from getting polio or taking it to their families. Every day at work they could look around at their patients and think, "There but for the grace of God go I—or my spouse or child."

In the late summer, they thought the epidemic was over. But then, Tisdale said, "we'd have a new case even more critically ill and more difficult to understand than the last." One of those complex, late cases was Alvin Levin, a lawyer from the nearby town of Lincoln. His wife, Betty, recalled that one of the doctors who helped put him in an iron lung was someone they had met through her job. The doctor broke down in tears when he looked into Alvin's face and realized it was someone he knew. The physicians were caring for their neighbors, friends, and colleagues from the same suburbs and towns they lived in. Tisdale remembered a bright psychiatry resident whom he'd known in the service who developed total body paralysis that summer. Another doctor took care of the wives of two colleagues; both women died.

Whitfield had a brief reprieve during that protracted polio season when a medical rotation sent him to the newborn unit in Providence for six weeks. "It was such a relief to get away from Boston and to be with happy mothers of new babies," he remembered. The rotation over, he went back to Massachusetts General, back to the polio. There, in mid-December he admitted yet another child with the disease.

RATHER THAN PROGRESSING in a steady rise or decline from year to year, the number of cases rolled up and down unpredictably, contributing to the fear and discouragement health officials and the public felt. Nineteen thousand people came down with polio in 1944 and 13,000 the next year, raising hopes that the viral disease was retreating. Then in 1946 more than 25,000 cases were reported, followed in 1947 by fewer than half that many. In the next polio season, however, the toll climbed to 28,000, nearly matching the bleak total for 1916. By midsummer of 1949, *Life* magazine reported that the 8,300 cases counted thus far for the year represented a 43 percent increase over the dismal 1948 figure. The writer announced wearily: "Polio seems more uncontrollable than ever."

The *New York Times*, the *Cleveland News*, and other daily newspapers around the country, along with local radio stations, reported daily tallies of the disease's somber march, often listing those who had been hospitalized or who had died from it. The lists grew longer as summer progressed, and people came to dread the roll call, fearing they would read or hear a name they knew. Despite the care with which health officials collected and newspapers reported the weekly, monthly, and yearly counts of polio cases, the numbers ultimately were unreliable. Mild cases went unreported, and odd illnesses symptomatically similar to polio—aseptic meningitis and Coxsackie viruses, for instance—were mistakenly included in the polio totals.

But the numbers were not what secured polio's place in the American psyche; no statistic can account for the awe and dread that surrounded polio. What nearly everyone who grew up in the polio years or who was rearing a child then remembers was the fear that hung like heat in the summer air.

The very mention of polio evoked disturbing images: rows and rows of iron lungs in big-city hospitals and game little children who, with their brace-supported legs, took lurching steps toward the arms of an encouraging nurse. The public couldn't help but be captured by photographs of the young man married in an iron lung, or of the three-year-old boy with a paralyzed arm entertaining his hospital friends by demonstrating his ability to pick up marbles and put them in a cup with his once-paralyzed toes. Cleveland residents picked up the *Cleveland News* on August 11, 1949, and saw the front-page headline "POLIO KILLS MOTHER OF STRICKEN CHILD; NEW FIGHT SPURRED." The newspaper account began: "The death today of an East Cleveland housewife, who contracted polio the day after her two-year-old daughter was taken to City Hospital with the same disease, aroused an entire neighborhood to caution in the face of an unseen killer." Three photographs allowed readers to stare into the faces of the besieged family. There was one of the smiling mother holding her handbag and wearing a fashionable hat, another of the grieving father clutching his seven-year-old son, and last, the still-hospitalized two-year-old daughter.

Despite the virulence of the disease and the intensity of the public's trepidation and concern, polio was never the leading childhood killer. Even during the worst epidemic years, far more children died or were crippled each year from accidents than from all childhood diseases together. A child under ten had only three chances in a thousand of becoming the victim of a severe attack of polio. The year my mother fell ill in Arizona, she was among only 701 reported polio cases in the state. Learning how few people actually had paralytic polio offered no comfort to me. And the statistics were no comfort to frantic parents of the 1940s and 1950s either. The one child in three hundred could be any child: the one down the street, the one down the hall. Parents could imagine warding off a life-threatening accident, but polio lurked, unseen, unfightable.

MOST OF THE TIME THE POLIOVIRUS goes no farther than the intestinal tract, where it might cause temporary discomfort, but no damage. The trouble comes when, for unknown reasons, the virus courses through the blood, finds the central nervous system, and destroys message-sending cells, sometimes causing permanent paralysis. "Even though this is estimated to occur in less than 3 to 4 percent of all poliovirus infections," wrote the medical historian John R. Paul, "the toll of disabled persons in a sizable epidemic can reach tremendous proportions."

Polio can circulate widely in a population, with a ratio of paralytic disease to inapparent infection as high as one to a thousand. That means that in 1952, the country's worst epidemic year, if the disease had been epidemic evenly throughout the country, as much as 40 percent of the U.S. population would have had polio. Medical researchers have long thought that most cases of polio passed unnoticed, having no symptoms at all, and that many others manifested in such a mild way, as sore throat, upset stomach, and "flu," that they were never diagnosed as polio. In fact, considering the almost universal spread of the virus during the prevaccine years, it's a wonder that any susceptible child in an epidemic area escaped infection for long. Just a few weeks before my mother was paralyzed, my brother's teacher sent him home from school with a 103-degree temperature that turned into a "bad cold." A week later I had a temperature of 104 degrees with no other symptoms, which the doctor attributed to an ear and throat infection. Did we actually have polio? Probably. Multiple cases in families were the rule, not the exception. I have a slight curve to my spine, something not uncommon and something that causes me no obvious difficulty, and I now suspect it to be a result of polio. How many of us were drawn to the brink of polio's chasm of crippling and death without even knowing we had been in danger?

After studying the 1944 Buffalo, New York, epidemic, scientists reported in 1946 to the American Medical Association a typical instance of how the disease crept insidiously through one family. In March, the family's seven-year-old girl had a headache and fever that lasted three days. Two weeks later her twin brother had a sore throat and was so ill his parents feared he was coming down with pneumonia. Then two more girls in the family, ages two and twelve, suffered bad colds. The mother and father had also spent three or four miserable days with headaches, sore throats, and diarrhea. Then on May 23, eleven weeks after the seven-year-old became ill, the four-year-old boy in the family developed paralytic polio. Researchers determined that all the other illnesses in the family from March to that day in May were mild, unrecognized cases of polio. The virus had been active in the house for eleven weeks before inexplicably ambushing the four-year-old.

THE HISTORY OF POLIO IS RIFE with misdiagnosis. My parents didn't suspect polio when my mother came down with a severe backache, because other reasonable explanations fit. The early stages could go on for days, with doctors telling patients they had the flu or pleurisy. Not suspecting polio, physicians prescribed codeine, penicillin, aspirin, and even antibiotics for their patients' aching bodies. Some doctors recommended rest for the unnamed symptoms, but many a doctor instructed mothers to encourage listless children to be busy and active. Often it wasn't until weakness turned to paralysis or breathing difficulty, or both, that doctors recognized polio.

The onset was bewildering for Betty Levin. Opening a drawer to get cutlery, she found she couldn't pick up the utensils, and the tips of her fingers were strangely sensitive. Her head and neck ached fiercely, and though the symptoms kept getting worse, she thought they must have something to do with her pregnancy, though this was her third. After a week of growing discomfort that was rapidly becoming agony, Betty's husband, Alvin, took her to the hospital. The doctor watched her walk in the examining room with her head bent forward at an odd angle from a stiffened neck and shuffling because her legs couldn't separate more than a couple of inches. He prescribed a painkiller and suggested she keep busy, then he shooed her away and chided her for malingering.

Once back home, Betty urged Alvin to go to work and called a neighbor to watch the children so she could go to bed and get some sleep. Later that day she was hospitalized in a delirium brought on by polio. Two weeks later when Alvin began to exhibit symptoms—fever, headache, neck ache, and an inability to urinate or bend over—he called a doctor, who told him not to worry. "Those are psycho-somatic," the doctor said, "because your wife had all the same symptoms." It took Alvin about an hour to realize the doctor was a fool. He called a friend to take him to a hospital, where he spent the next year and a half before being discharged as a quadriplegic.

Although some doctors were careless or cruel, even the most well-meaning and well-trained ones could be deceived by the vague and varied ways polio presented itself. Late one night during the summer of 1955 in the emergency room at Massachusetts General, Thomas Whitfield admitted a child with paralysis of an eye muscle, a condition he knew could come with ear infection. He sat exhausted from a long shift, thinking about the child and suddenly wondered whether she had polio showing up only as eye-muscle paralysis. He immediately ordered a spinal tap that confirmed polio, and she was moved to the floor for contagious diseases. The doctor suffered, he told me, knowing that by admitting her first to the regular hospital he had risked exposing others to the disease.

Polio varies widely not only in its intensity but in its lasting effects. Children can hover near death fully paralyzed and recover completely, or they can be left with paralysis ranging from the inconvenient to the tragic. Infectious disease specialists working in the 1950s saw many more deaths from measles than from polio, but measles did not terrify parents as did polio, which could end forever a child's running and jumping. Polio sometimes left peculiar, life-changing disabilities. It struck one boy in July 1951 and paralyzed his throat and neck, rendering him unable to support his head or swallow. He chewed his food by using his hand to move his jaw. And, of course, polio landed many people in an iron lung. About half the time, whatever muscle weakness polio brought on subsided within six months or so, yet no one looking at two new polio victims could say what the outcome for each might be. Polio could attack two people standing side by side, two brothers, even, and the outcome for each could be entirely different.

James and William Warwick, brothers who grew up in Massachusetts, received college degrees in the spring of 1955—a master's for James and a bachelor's for William. Both brothers signed teaching contracts for the school year beginning in September. James was to teach at a small college in upstate New York; Bill, at a high school in Hingham, Massachusetts. James spent the summer at leisure, taking his veteran's pay and waiting for his pregnant wife to deliver their first child. Bill, a year and a half younger at age twenty-two was already the father of two sons, and worked two jobs. In early September, the two men, who were close to each other, loaded a rental truck, and James, with his wife and infant, set out for New York. The first night, James was sick; chills kept him under layers of blankets, as he sipped hot tea at the motel. The next morning he was fine, and the family headed north again. A day later they arrived in Potsdam. As they were unpacking, they received a telegram from his mother saying that Bill was in an iron lung with polio and probably would not live.

Did James have polio also? If so, the result was one bad night, while his brother spent the next twenty-plus years as a quadriplegic.

THROUGH THE MANY LONG YEARS of polio's reign, study, testing, and observation revealed many characteristics of the disease. Unaccountably, it affects boys more severely than girls, stress increases a person's susceptibility, and more pregnant than nonpregnant women suffer the paralytic form of the disease. Many adults, both victims and family members of victims, like Martha Hoover, could look at their activities over the days preceding their illnesses and wonder whether they could have done something different that would have given them the power to shake off the disease. Betty Levin had been hospitalized for two weeks when her husband, Alvin, began exhibiting symptoms. He had, as she said, "done everything wrong." Instead of resting completely once she came down with polio, in hopes of lessening the impact in case he also got it, he did what most conscientious husbands and fathers would have done: he took care of their two young children by day and did his job at night. And he came down with a case of the disease that rendered him paralyzed for life. Betty eventually recovered completely.

Although the word *stress* was never used then, it seemed to contribute to susceptibility. Mary Bready of Baltimore was one of twelve adult patients at a children's hospital in 1952, and half of them, including her, had moved into new houses within the month or so before the onset of polio. My mother also had been preparing for a move when she became ill, and I wonder now whether the combination of physical exhaustion and emotional strain contributed to the severity of her case.

Much of the apprehension surrounding polio came from the unknown. Despite rigorous research, nothing could tell public health authorities where the next polio outbreak might occur—and even if they had known, they could not have stopped it. No one knew how many kinds of polio there were, and treatment was long a matter of controversy. In 1949 one *Saturday Evening Post* writer noted that scientists did not understand "the hidden battle that goes on between the nerve cells and the polio virus." In ignorance, the writer explained, "Even now they cannot watch the contest in a human patient, because the nerves are buried in the flesh, and the flesh is too tender to permit much investigative probing."

Most frightening of all, no one knew how you got it. Did you breathe it in, swallow it in contaminated milk, drink it down at a public fountain, or get it from flies on your picnic lunch? The most innocent activity, it seemed, could condemn you to a lifetime in braces or, worse, closed into an iron lung. The lack of specific, reliable information about how the virus spread frustrated and scared health officials, physicians, scientists, politicians and, certainly, the public.

Throughout the first half of this century, scientists worked diligently, though not always effectively, to solve the mystery of polio's transmission. In the thirties some widely published accounts made popular the notion that the virus invaded through the nerves of smell. Years before, in 1910, a scientist who transmitted the disease to monkeys by rubbing the virus into their nose membranes first suggested the theory. As the years went on and no better idea about how one got polio was advanced, the theory took on importance. In 1936, the physician Charles Armstrong, with the U.S. Public Health Service, decided that coating the olfactory nerves would block the entry of the poliovirus. He sprayed a picric acid and alum solution into the noses of forty-six hundred Alabamians, to no good end. Another doctor, Edwin Schultz of Stanford, thought the compound zinc sulfate could do the job better. He also thought the patient's sense of smell had to be deadened in order for the preventive treatment to take effect. In 1937 he sprayed the noses of five thousand children in Toronto, Canada, with the only result being that a few permanently lost their sense of smell.

By the late thirties scientists knew polio was an acute viral disease that attacked the nervous system. They knew that the virus left the body through the bowels and the saliva, but they did not know how long people with inapparent cases of nonparalytic polio harbored the infection. They had seen the poliovirus through the electron microscope, but they still didn't know how it traveled from person to person. That, of course, didn't stop them from speculating. Rats, moles, and household pets were implicated. Public toilets and drinking fountains were suspected. Some scientists thought hair, skin, eye color, and diet contributed to a person's susceptibility. Others pointed the finger at a recessive gene; while others identified sore throats and sinus trouble as the factors that could predispose one to polio. Droplets in the air were thought to carry polio through coughs, sneezes, and breath to new victims; food, milk, and water, it was believed, could be contaminated with polio and ingested. One epidemiologist studying polio for the NFIP in 1946 reported that sewage waters used to irrigate truck farms in Denver contained the virus and that his studies had revealed outbreaks of polio in Florida and Arkansas following shipments of Denver truck-garden vegetables. The link, however, could have been merely coincidental, he noted. But it was the kind of news that set mothers to scrubbing and boiling vegetables.

Scientists worked for decades to link poliomyelitis with flies. When, at the turn of the century, yellow fever was found to be carried by mosquitoes, speculation rose about the role of insects in the spread of other diseases. By 1938, knowing that polio affected the intestines and that infected people shed the virus in their stools, scientists deduced that flies, especially the feces-eating types, could carry the virus to food and people.

Then three laboratories, including the Yale Poliomyelitis Unit, isolated the virus in several types of common flies in epidemic areas in the summer and fall of 1941. Some thought it was the breakthrough scientists had dreamed of. If flies could be eliminated, then perhaps so could polio epidemics.

About the same time, the chemical insecticide DDT was introduced. Used mainly in areas of the South Pacific islands to protect armed forces from malaria-infected mosquitoes, with almost miraculous results, DDT seemed to be the magic potion that could control all insect pests. Knowing that flies carried polio and that DDT could eliminate flies, the next steps, according to the physician John R. Paul, a medical historian and former member of the Yale Poliomyelitis team, seemed simple. They weren't.

The Yale Unit, working with the U.S. Public Health Service, began controlled experiments to try to eliminate flies from certain areas. They successfully reduced the number of flies in Savannah, Georgia, and Paterson, New Jersey, but they saw no reduction in polio cases—probably, they thought, because there was too little polio there. What they needed for a true experiment was some place with a full-blown epidemic going. They found it in Rockford, Illinois, in the summer of 1945.

What the experimenters did not account for in their preparations was the hysteria that surrounded polio epidemics. Expecting to carry out their tests under carefully controlled, even secret conditions, they instead found themselves the subject of blaring headlines. Newspaper reporters got wind that Rockford was being considered for the experiments and rashly announced that spraying the area with insecticide was the one thing that could save the residents from the scourge of polio.

On the first day of spraying, two-inch-high newspaper headlines screamed: "PROFESSOR EXPECTED TO BOARD MERCY PLANE AT NOON TODAY." It was August 18, 1945, just days after the bombing of Hiroshima, and one newspaper declared with its headline: "PREVENTATIVE SPRAYING FOR POLIO AS IMPORTANT TO ROCKFORD AS THE ATOMIC BOMB." Eleven men sprayed, from the air and on the ground, for six days. The result: a temporary reduction of flies, but no halt in the polio epidemic. The Yale team made no more attempts to experiment with fly abatement, and their theory went the way of nasal sprays.

Ultimately, scientists determined that flies didn't play a major role in spreading the virus, at least in communities where sanitation was adequate. But that news wasn't widely known, and the general public, at least, continued to fear flies during polio summers. In light of what we know now about DDT, we can only be grateful that the powerful, highly toxic chemical failed to have an impact on polio epidemics. Had it shown even a hint of success, the insecticide surely would have been applied wholesale.

CURRENT UNDERSTANDING is that polio, like other gastro-intestinal diseases, spreads by personal contact, most commonly through the mouth, with an already infected person. I've tried to imagine what it must have been like then to be a parent, living in a pristine suburb of Houston, a homogeneous mill town on the banks of a New England river, or a fourth-floor walk-up apartment on Chicago's South Side, with another summer approaching, knowing there was an unseen contagion that could invade my home, my child—a contagion that perhaps could be picked up as a result of a sneeze on a bus or a bite of food. And no scientist or doctor could say for sure what I should do to protect my family.

Polio's association with summer, an oddity still unexplained, contributed to its mystique. The time when children and families were otherwise most healthy and carefree came to be a time of sickness and dread. No one knew then nor knows now why polio erupted in the summertime, though clearly it did. The polio season, like the ripening of crops, began in the South in the early spring and spread northward through the summer. Doctors had long suspected that epidemics could be well under way before paralytic cases showed up, but scientists were confused about why, if polio was silently active in communities for months, the paralytic symptoms seemed to appear only in the summer months. Researchers studying epidemics in Chicago and Buffalo in the forties offered several theories. They suggested that polio flared in summertime because of more numerous and widespread human contacts, or because physical fatigue during the incubation period encouraged paralysis, and children exercise more vigorously in the summer. Or perhaps it was because the virus survived more easily in sunshine and heat than in cold. The public devised its own theories as well. Anything associated with summer—exposure to the sun and swimming, even the consumption of cola drinks—drew suspicion.

The implicit threat of disease curtailed summer pleasures for the children of the polio years. Mothers and fathers, once tolerant of neighborhood evening games of kick-the-can, of long afternoons spent at the baseball field, matinee movies, or swimming pools, now were heard to say to their protesting children, "Do you want to spend the rest of your life in an iron lung?" Alex Coffin, who was born in 1936, remembers that the small North Carolina textile town of about seven thousand where he grew up suffered no polio cases, but fear of the disease "put a crimp" in his playtime. A drainage ditch less than a foot wide divided his family's yard from that of the next-door neighbors, and the boys who lived in those houses had to play with the ditch between them rather than venture into each other's yards. A friend of mine, born in 1950 and reared in Chicago, remembers sitting on the shore of Lake Michigan, sweating in the summer heat but forbidden to go in the water because a child had been stricken with polio after swimming there. She recalls trying to picture what this thing called polio looked like, as she stared into the water, hoping for a glimpse of the dreaded, fascinating ogre.

Other children who were forbidden to congregate spent their summers reading, playing card games, and following other solitary pursuits. "I don't remember chafing unduly," remembers one such confined child of the forties, "for none of us wanted to contract polio."

Local newspapers and radios pitched in with efforts to entertain children who were confined to their backyards, as in 1946 when Minneapolis was hit with an epidemic. The *Minneapolis Daily Times* ran a full page titled: "Hey, Gang! Have FUN at Home. Just Look at These Swell Games You Can Play in Your Own Neighborhood." Radio stations scheduled special programs, including the comedian Bob Hope in "I Never Left Home." In its effort to keep children home during the epidemic, the city forbade children under fifteen in movie theaters, churches, Sunday schools, youth centers, and amusement parks. The Masons canceled picnics. A synagogue canceled its ice cream social and auction sale. The swimming beaches on those hot summer afternoons remained as empty as classrooms.

The question of whether children were safe at summer camp or not made for much parental discussion and anxiety. Some parents sent their children to camp, thinking that they were protecting them from exposure; others kept theirs home for the same reason. Some camps closed because children came down with polio. Others coped by dispensing large, dark-colored vitamins, by posting warnings in the bathrooms about hand washing, and by keeping a sharp eye for sore throats, lassitude, pains, and stiffness in campers. They banished all visitors or divided them from campers with a wide corridor set off by ropes.

As did many other summer camps, Camp Catawba, near Blowing Rock, North Carolina, enforced partial or full quarantines for its young male campers in order to avoid contact with the outside world during the state's epidemic years. Counselors seldom went into town in the evenings or on their days off. Visitors to the camp and the boys themselves endured cleansing rituals, and campers stayed away from the local annual horse show. The camp's founder told parents of her concern and offered her reassurances in letters sent home to them:

> August 1, 1948. Dear Parents: I know perfectly well that all of you are following with anxiety the newspaper reports on the polio epidemic in this state. Yet keep in mind: your children are in the safest place and the most complete isolation on our hilltop. We receive reports and advice from the State Board of Health twice a week. We take all possible precautions such as: mopping, spraying, dish washing with disinfectants; no visits of the boys in Blowing Rock; no visitors on camp grounds; every adult who has been to the village gargles and washes before coming in contact with the children.

> August 8, 1948. Dear Parents: The responsibility for the boys is weighing heavily on us these days. I can absolutely reassure you about their safety while they are at

camp. It seems too early to worry about their trip home. If the epidemic should not have died down until then we may have to have them go back from another railroad station so as to avoid infected areas.

The boys from Camp Catawba ultimately avoided the train—and polio—altogether that summer. The camp rented a school bus and drove them home north along the Blue Ridge Parkway. The following summer when polio struck New York, the camp extended its season an extra week so that the boys could avoid the afflicted city a bit longer.

IN ANY ONGOING EPIDEMIC THAT HAS NO CURE and no immediate prospect for vaccine, as with AIDS today, prevention becomes the primary focus for the public. And so parents paid attention to the guidelines set out in NFIP brochures, which directed them to give children plenty of fresh air: avoid the crowds of trains, buses, boats, beaches, and theaters; and prevent "too strenuous play, late hours, irregular schedules"—all of which were seen as "possible invitations to attack by polio." When *Life* magazine listed polio "hazards to avoid," parents took note that "raw milk may be contaminated by insects or by germs out of the air" and that "food should be covered." Following guidelines set out by the NFIP, newspapers and magazines told parents they should make sure their children had plenty of fresh air and adequate diets. Americans were told to wash their hands before eating or handling food, to eat at home instead of at restaurants, to keep their garbage well covered, and to screen their houses against flies and mosquitoes. Families were cautioned against travel, for fear they would take polio from one area to another or unnecessarily risk entering an epidemic area. Parents were told to teach their children to keep their fingers out of their mouths and "not to swap pencils, whistles, apples, lollypops or any other object they are likely to put in their mouths," and to wash their hands before meals.

Experts repeatedly cautioned parents not to allow their children to become fatigued, because it was thought then, and is known now to be so, that children who engaged in strenuous exercise were more apt to get the disease and to get more serious cases than those who were kept quiet. After observing that vigorous activity often preceded severe paralysis, a neurologist in Oxford, England, was convinced that extreme physical exertion in the first critical days before any paralysis "is almost suicidal, while the continuance of even average physical activity is dangerous." It was thought, as the *Saturday Evening Post* reported in 1949, that pregnancy and even daily routines "may [have made] the embattled nerve cells more vulnerable and hinder[ed] their recovery."

One NFIP epidemiologist further speculated that leg exercise, such as long bicycle rides, could mean a child would be affected in the legs if he soon contracted polio or was in the latent stage of the disease at the time, and that strenuous arm use could leave those limbs vulnerable to attack. In an effort to comply with the warnings against exhaustion, many children were put to bed before dark in the summer and required to interrupt their roller skating or ball playing for afternoon naps.

In the early forties researchers reasserted an earlier observation that children who had had recent tonsillectomies were prone to contracting polio. The medical literature reported dramatic and tragic stories of polio following tonsil operations, perhaps because the poliovirus, often present in the pharynx during epidemics, made its way quickly through the nerve endings exposed by surgery to the central nervous system. That news put a halt to many a grade-school child's scheduled operation. The physician for Frances Billings, now Frances Finke, and her family knew of the association with tonsillectomies in 1944, but because the teen had been plagued with severe sore throats through several winters, he determined she should have the operation. To be safe, he scheduled her surgery for November, long after freezing temperatures had come to their Wisconsin community, when, presumably, the cold would have killed off the "polio germ." On December 1, 1944, still recovering from the tonsillectomy, Frances was hospitalized with a devastating case of polio. The doctor wept when he got the news.

ALWAYS, MISINFORMATION CIRCULATED along with news of the latest scientific discoveries. Little of what was known about polio provided any help or comfort, leading people to clutch at whatever clue might provide protection. Often the few facts that were clear to those scientists studying the disease did not reach the public or even health-care providers with any reliability. In 1949, John A. Toomey, the head of the department of contagious disease at City Hospital in Cleveland and someone identified as a "widely known authority" in the *Cleveland Plain Dealer*, was quoted as saying that polio was "relatively new and increasing," unlike influenza, which dated back to biblical times. He also said the disease was not yet proved to be contagious and that its symptoms were "not too well defined." He continued, "But if an individual has trouble with his throat—particularly his throat muscles—he very likely has polio." The well-intentioned, but not particularly well-informed, doctor also advised readers that if polio was to be prevented, "the bowels must be kept open."

Confronted throughout the polio years with reams of information—much of it conflicting, little of it reassuring—parents often devised their own theories about how people caught polio and how they could ward it off. Mothers boiled dishes, cautioned their children away from public drinking fountains, and wiped every surface with alcohol. They told their children ice cream could harbor polio germs. Noticing that each year polio flared at the same time that peaches came on the market, they banished the fruit from their homes. Some switched to canned peaches, pears, and applesauce while the season's new fruit hung on the trees. Parents relentlessly discouraged flies, years after the Yale experiment had shown that flies were not the problem. When the newspapers started predicting an epidemic year in the spring, they pulled their children out of school. And if summer did bring an epidemic, schools sometimes opened late, or parents kept their children home.

Grandmothers fashioned "acidify bags," muslin pouches holding a piece of alum, and pinned them to children's underwear, certain it held the protective magic youngsters needed. Others put their faith in camphor. One mother insisted her two small sons wear white cotton gloves in movie theaters. (They were allowed to wait until the hall went dark before slipping on their protection against what their mother called "the deadly, and easily spread germ.")

Mothers throughout the country periodically performed a widely known "polio test" on their children, particularly if they complained in the least about not feeling well. Children were to sit up straight and put their chins to their chests. If there was any pain, polio was suspected. One girl and her sister were periodically put through this test until one day it hurt for her to bend her head. She had a mild case that left her right calf weak. Mary Bready, a young mother in Baltimore, discovered she had polio in the summer of 1952, when, after enduring days of ill health, she was struggling up the stairs to lie down on her bed and suddenly remembered to check for polio. Her head wouldn't bend at all.

Parents often misconstrued advice from the NFIP and doctors. Hearing that travel was inadvisable, one family left the youngest child at home, thinking she was most vulnerable to polio, and took her older brothers on a vacation. And everyone, it seems, had his or her own theory about water and swimming. Mothers cautioned their children to stay away from oil-skimmed dirty water in the streets and to avoid swimming in "stirred-up," clouded water. Cold water was especially feared, probably because it was common knowledge that on the day FDR had fallen ill, he had taken a swim in the icy bay near his summer home. Thus, city parents made their children resist the icy flowing water of "fireplug" showers on hot summer days. Other parents decided that public swimming pools were off limits, but that swimming holes in woodland creeks were safe. And in communities around the country, popular swimming sites were closed down. During the epidemic in Hickory, North Carolina, a boy biked out to Lake Hickory one hot summer afternoon and found the popular recreation area deserted. The Boy Scout cabin on the lake stood empty; a popular beach and a nearby restaurant languished, and the water's surface lay undisturbed. "Even boaters dared not risk polio," he remembered.

From the moment cases began to be listed in the Rockford, Illinois, newspapers, eleven-year-old Patricia Altenberg Lovett, an only child, wasn't allowed even to venture into the yard. No bus rides into town to see movies, no trips to the library, no wanderings through the aisles of the Woolworth store, no walks to the drugstore with her girlfriends for an ice cream cone during that summer of 1945. To keep the girl busy, Patricia's mother made frequent trips downtown to collect paper dolls and books to bring home. Patricia's biggest disappointment, however, was missing the home games of the Rockford Peaches, the All-American girls' baseball team. Her parents took turns going to games so they could give her reports.

In August that summer, Japan surrendered in the Pacific and World War II ended. The whistles blew at the factories not far from where the family lived, and car horns sounded as those fortunate few with gasoline drove around celebrating. Patricia missed the whole thing. She longed to go down into the center of Rockford and join the celebrating throngs. But she stayed home, and that's where she was when school began in September. Her parents were convinced that the epidemic would spread faster and the lists of ill and dead would grown longer once the children convened for classes. Two weeks into the school year, that had not happened, and so Patricia entered sixth grade. When her first day of school finally arrived, she was welcomed with hand clapping and joy by her classmates, who had saved her a seat in the middle of the classroom.

Little wonder parents sometimes responded to epidemics in extreme ways. The NFIP kept awareness of polio high, and then tried to calm the fears it raised. A 1947 brochure directed at parents said, "Carry on your normal activities. Remember, most patients get well, and with good care the majority recover without crippling. Your fear or panic will only make it harder for your children." The brochure went on to assure parents that polio broke out infrequently and attacked few people, and that deformities could be prevented and lessened by prompt, complete, and "sometimes prolonged" medical care. But who can blame parents for not being reassured by such pronouncements from the same people who, in their fund-raising efforts, blanketed the country with heart-tugging pictures of crippled children.

The press carried a similar set of contradictory messages, one day reporting that orange juice could cause polio and the next running such articles as "Let's Be Sane about Polio," as *Parents* magazine did in 1953. One magazine called polio a "Hopeless Disease," while also offering vitamin E as a possible cure. In August 1949, the *Cleve-land Plain Dealer* reported that the year-to-date tally of polio cases was not at an epidemic level, but also said that the disease had "extended its grip on Ohio." Nonetheless, the state fair was going on as sched-uled. What was a parent to think if the disease held a "grip" on the state? Did responsible parents take their children to the state fair?

CONTRIBUTING TO ITS SOCIAL IMPACT was polio's coinci-dence with the postwar baby boom. Between 1947 and 1953 a new generation of parents bore babies at a rate that increased the popula-tion of the United States more than it had grown from 1917 to 1947. In the postwar decade, the United States was a nation of mostly middle-class parents, ones who for the first time in history had the money and the leisure to be vitally interested in the well-being of their children. For this first wave of parents nurtured on the advice of the pediatrician Benjamin Spock, having children became a self-conscious act, something to do well and to read about, think about, and talk about. And for many women, who had held down jobs dur-ing the war and were now enveloped in domesticity, it was the only thing they had to do. Into this buoyant postwar era came a fearsome disease to haunt their lives and to help spoil for those young parents the idealized notion of what family life would be. Polio was a crack in the fantasy. Thinking of his paralyzed six-year-old son, one father in the fifties spoke of the altered future: "We tell ourselves, 'My boy, I can see in him possibilities untold.' . . . Polio kills that. It stops the dream."

Polio created an epidemic of fear unlike any other in modern times. For every family struck, someone asked silently, if not aloud, "*Why us? Why me?*" Any serious misfortune can leave a victim searching for answers and explanations, but polio was peculiarly un-yielding to accountability. The disease attacked everyone's sense of fairness and muddied their notion of justice. Fred Davis, a sociologist at the University of California Medical Center at San Francisco, wrote about children crippled by polio and asserted that getting polio was "a kind of discriminatory barrier in the attainment of important social values; in short, it was 'unAmerican.' " In polio epidemics, rewards and punishments were dispensed with a random, devastating hand. Parents of stricken children, Davis found, asked themselves what they had done wrong, for surely they had done something; according to the value system in this country, misfortune isn't supposed to touch those who take precautions.

The disease stood as an ominous reminder that Americans were still vulnerable to the forces of nature, that scientists couldn't put everything right. Americans had conquered other diseases and had created the world's best technology, yet polio defied everyone's best efforts. No one knew how to prevent it or to lessen one's risks. Throughout the epidemic years parents in stricken communities did everything possible, from the mundane to the extreme, to prevent their children from contracting the disease. Still, children—and adults—got polio.

CHAPTER THREE

Waiting

In the two days it took polio to render Mother helpless, our precious, unexceptional life of desert picnics, unpaid bills, and supper at the kitchen table vanished. Unintentionally, unwillingly we became the exception. The disease overwhelmed her—and everyone else in our family—with its swift capture. One day she was our familiar, loving mother grown tired and achy. Two days later, without warning, she was transformed, trapped in a body that didn't function, close to death, more a stranger, even to herself, than our cherished Virginia. While my father, grandparents, brother, and I stood helpless, Mother descended into an abyss of physical and mental suffering.

When I set out to discover what I could about the disease that took her, I knew little about the woman who was my mother—very little, even, of the most basic facts about my family background. And I had gone thirty-seven years into my life without realizing how odd the gaps in my knowledge were. Until 1987 when I began the slow journey to uncover her history and mine, I couldn't have said the names of my father's parents. I didn't know in what year my parents were born, nor in what house our family lived when I came into the world. And as for the particulars of polio itself, I knew none, for in the years after my mother's illness and death the disease had disappeared from public awareness, as well as from my family's consciousness.

IN FEBRUARY 1990, I bought and moved into a little Victorian house set against the mountains that provide a backdrop to Boulder, my parents' and my hometown. I hadn't lived there since 1971 when I graduated from the University of Colorado, married, and moved away. I was twenty-two then and already had left Boulder three times, only to go back. Whether I was taken away as a child or went voluntarily as an adult, I returned, unconsciously echoing the pattern of my mother's life. If anytime from 1971 until 1987 someone had suggested that my longing for Colorado, which gently nagged my years in Kansas City, New York, and San Francisco, had anything to do with my mother, I would have said, "Nonsense." I felt in control of my ambitions and emotions—sure, most of all, that whatever had happened to my mother had no significance in my life.

My return to Boulder after nearly twenty years away, however, was a step in the journey I had begun toward finding her, though just how I wasn't sure. All I knew at the time was that I was newly divorced, weary of city life, and yearning for connection, continuity, and family, and that I needed a home. I began to make one for myself, starting with the externals: the move to Boulder to a house of my own, one with bookshelves, a fireplace, a second story, and a garden. And then, two months after moving in, a hundred feet from my back door, an airplane dropped from a Sunday morning sky, crashed in the alley behind my house, and killed the pilot and his passenger. The explosion, which left nothing but small, unrecognizable pieces of the plane, ignited a fire that burned a neighbor's house to the ground, along with half a dozen garages and sheds lining the alley. Anything, *anything* can happen, it told me—a reminder of the unconscious awareness I'd gained at age four, when an unforeseeable disaster had taken my mother. When the plane crashed, it sounded a note that harmonized with the disaster of my early life.

The day after the crash, on the evening news, my sooty but otherwise undamaged car in its partly charred garage flashed on the television screen. The camera zoomed close to show my California license plates. The reporter noted that I had just moved from San Francisco, where the 7.1 earthquake of the previous fall had stunned that city. What the reporter didn't say was that my apartment had been in the Marina District, where, a block away, a blaze sparked by the earthquake had burned for five hours, killing some of my neighbors. Weeks later when I left San Francisco for my already planned move to Colorado, I packed, along with my household belongings, a fresh awareness of life's fragility and unpredictability. In leaving, I carried a dim sense of relief, of good fortune as I turned my back on the rubble of my first marriage and my neighborhood. And then, not expecting—as none of us ever do—further evidence of the arbitrary nature of life, I found it again in my Colorado garden.

These odd disasters coming so close together compelled me to see again, this time with knowledge, not merely awareness, the truth that life's surprises have no limits. I knew these events weren't personal in the sense that I had not caused them nor had they, any more than my mother's illness, occurred in order to teach me something. But they were personal in that they happened in my life, and each, for a time, deeply disturbed me and disrupted my days. Believing that wisdom reveals itself in our responses to the random events that occur in and around our lives, I wanted to pay attention this time, to listen to the sounds of these events and not just let them tumble around me. I wanted to take from these miseries a truth. And what I took was the truth that if anything can happen, then maybe even what seemed the most impossible occurrence of all could transpire: that I might come to understand my past, that I might find my mother in that discovery, and that from it all I might create my place in a family again. Maybe *that* kind of anything could happen, too.

DRIVEN TO KNOW WHAT my mother experienced while stranded in her broken body, I plunged into reading accounts of other profoundly affected polio victims, only to recoil, repeatedly, as I discovered how dreadful polio could be. I couldn't separate those stories from my mother, and in reading each one, I unwillingly substituted Mother for each severe case. In his memoir, Robert F. Hall, who contracted polio in 1949 just as he graduated from Yale, recounted the sounds he and his hospital roommates overheard across the hallway as a mother of three died of bulbar polio. Her twin, the mother of four children, had died five days earlier:

She saw what had happened to her sister in the same room and now she was taking the same course. Bed tilted up in the air, head down and oxygen bubbling life into her through the green tube in her nose.

The night shift came on, and the quiet . . . accentuated the activity and sounds in her room. . . . The coughing became weaker. After gargling on her phlegm for a while, she began to choke. We cleared our own throats. . . . [I]t was not long before she began to cry out in a faint voice, "Help. Oh, please won't someone help me? Please help me. Please." . . . We traced the progress of the bulbar's attack at the base of her brain as the throat muscles collapsed. Her attempt to breathe, her dry coughs and the suction machine's hissing all became a conglomeration of sputtering sounds that made my stomach squirm and my heart ache. . . . As morning passed, her throat muscles were entirely gone and her breathing was cut off. Her strength was sapped from the battle through the night. . . . She went quickly; by afternoon, she was in the iron lung and she died the next morning. Then followed the sickening smell of the disinfectant.

No one can tell me for certain, but I can guess that Mother's first night passed in much the same way, with the notable exception that she survived.

ONCE TUCKED INTO THE COCOON of her iron lung, Mother breathed. She had survived the initial crisis, but death stalked her. My grandparents stayed at a nearby motel and visited daily, along with my father. Coming out of the hospital in the 100-degree and hotter sunshine, my grandmother remembers going to the car and being unable to touch the steering wheel. She wrapped the blazing plastic in a cloth and drove away to pass the sweltering hours until she could visit again. Although not a record-setting summer, the temperatures stayed high through Mother's acutely critical weeks. My grandmother has always hated Arizona for its heat and its memories.

As with many victims of severe cases, Mother's early months, my father tells me, were a blur of medical crisis upon crisis. She couldn't cough or sneeze or blow her nose, so a simple cold threatened her life more than once. Without her medical records, which Phoenix Memorial Hospital tells me no longer exist, I'll never know for certain what specific miseries Mother suffered, but I know that other patients similarly weakened fought pneumonia, as well as ear and other infections, and that the unspeakable pain of polio sometimes went on for weeks. I know from my father that Mother continued precariously ill through the summer, making her care an around-the-clock task.

Sometime during those first days she became aware of the contraption that held her. Most everyone who ended up in iron lungs had seen them only in black-and-white newspaper photos and on newsreels and so were surprised at some being mustard-colored, others muddy green. Some children, like the nine-year-old New York City girl Sharon Stern, knew little of iron lungs before entering one. Having been rushed in an ambulance from one hospital to another, she was unconscious, probably from lack of oxygen, when placed in her tank. She woke later with "a huge disk around [her] neck and shoulders." She looked up at the nurse and said, "I can't believe I slept in this thing. Can you take it off?" When her mother came to see her, Sharon told her, too, that she had slept in the thing and wanted it taken away. She was in the tank for weeks without knowing what it looked like, and then one day she saw one in a mirror when it was wheeled past her doorway.

Mostly, though, iron-lung patients were surprised by the noise, the powerful whooshing bellows and maddeningly rhythmic squeaks and whines of the machine. The father of Frances Billings Finke, the young girl from Wisconsin, found the suction of the iron lung that held her to be similar to the windshield wipers on his car. "That memory haunted him," she told me, "so he only used his wipers for big rains after that." The presence of iron lungs, with their noise and implications, weighed on all patients confined on those wards. Sid Moody, who came down with polio in the summer of 1949 after his junior year at Williams College, told me of his time confined in New York Hospital in a room of four men and boys, one in an iron lung. "Sleeping in a room with an iron lung is not easy, physically and psychologically," he recalled. "Part of you is alert to any break in the clanking rhythm which might jeopardize the life of someone now your friend. Another part of you wants to turn the damn thing off so you can sleep."

Ideally, hospitals provided each iron lung patient a single nurse, but few hospitals could manage that, especially during epidemics. At a Michigan hospital in the late forties, the nurse Ruth Hazen had charge of two respirator patients at a time. Because many chores, particularly bathing and changing sheets inside the tanks, required two people, the nurses teamed up, leaving three patients alone while they worked on one. When possible, nurses took patients out of their iron lungs for bathing and cleaning. Some could last a minute or two breathing with, perhaps, a single operative chest muscle or one side of the diaphragm, but even so, Hazen remembers, "some became very agitated and frightened so that this operation had to be done at top speed. . . . As the patients began to trust that we were not going to prolong their solo breathing, they were able to relax and breathe alone for longer periods of time. We liked to return them to the respirator before they were desperate. We timed and noted their 'out' very carefully, as this was an indication of their progress." Mother had no "out" time, because she couldn't breathe at all unassisted. Nurses stood on each side of her tank and changed the sheets through the armhole vents. "This was a difficult maneuver," said Hazen, "and not too satisfactory in terms of removing wrinkles in the sheets, but we became fairly proficient, especially as the team learned each other's pace."

Like Mother, Louis Sternburg, a young father and salesman in New England when he came down with polio, couldn't breathe outside his iron lung and required constant care. He recorded that early period of illness in a memoir he wrote with his wife Dorothy Sternburg: "As I slid in and out of comas, the nurses stuffed wadding around me and the lung got more and more unsanitary. I could feel wet and dirty, but as my head was outside the lung, I couldn't smell much." He had to be removed from the lung periodically for thorough cleaning, because the filth bred bedsores. To perform the chore, nurses loosened the clamps that sealed the machine at his head and wheeled him on his cot away from the iron cylinder, while an anesthesiologist kept him alive with "bag breathing," a temporary measure that involved attaching an oxygen line to the tracheotomy tube. The doctor then rhythmically squeezed a bag on the oxygen line, forcing air into the lungs. To clean him, nurses rolled him to one side, with the bag breathing going on, which terrified and disoriented him.

FOR THE DAY UPON DAY that turned to weeks and months, no one could say what would become of Mother. Then, as now, once the polio attack had begun, doctors had no way of arresting or lessening the severity of the virus's effects. Nor could they treat the destroyed cells to give them back their power. Nor could physicians measure the extent of the cells' damage except by looking to the muscles themselves and judging their tone, strength, and flaccidity. Fred Davis, who studied recovering polio patients, labeled that early period, while the virus did its voracious work and doctors tried to assess the damage, the "inventory stage" of the crisis.

Our family lived in suspension, waiting for news, for signs of hope, but there were few for Mother. She could move little more than her eyes, and she remained entirely dependent on her iron tomb for breath. Diminished in every way by illness, her face took on a detached, vacant expression; her body, visible only through the portholes of her tank, shrank from her usual 120 pounds on her five-foot, seven-inch frame to 90 pounds. Respiratory victims commonly wasted away to skin-covered bones. Within weeks a ten-year-old girl fell to the weight of a three- or four-year-old. A strong teenage boy lost half his 140 pounds in seven weeks. Paralyzed muscles lost tone and became flaccid; with severe damage they further degenerated through shrinkage and atrophy. Eating lost its appeal when bowels could no longer handle waste easily. I saw a photograph of a nurse, holding a tray heavy with dishes of food and a pint-sized milk bottle, standing at the head of a woman in an iron lung. The woman smiled, the nurse smiled. Yet as I stared at the photograph, I began to see a ludicrousness in it, to see how formidable the simple task of eating would have been for that supine woman. I lay on my back myself to try swallowing, without gravity to drop the bites into my stomach. Food fell to the back of my throat and down the side of my face.

Arnold Beisser, a recent graduate of Stanford University Medical School and a national tennis champion when he got polio in 1950, was in an iron lung from the first moments of his illness. Years later he wrote: "Lying immobile on my back, I found that everything looked big and menacing. Even familiar things seemed strange. The taste of food that I had once enjoyed seemed different when it came at me from the hand of another, swooping down from above. I ate very little." Victims lay wasting away, yet heavy in their immobility.

In her iron lung, Mother had to relearn the most basic of functions: breathing, eating, moving bowels, and urinating. One of the first skills most tank patients learned, however, was to summon help. Some clacked their teeth together; some made a popping sound with their lips. But most compressed and released air between the tongue and cheek to create a clicking sound like that used in urging a horse to go forward. They used the sound to signal for help if something happened to disable the respirator (and thus cut off the air they needed for speaking) or if tracheotomies made speech impossible. Frantic clicking, loud enough to be heard even by nurses tending to other patients at a distance, came from patients suffering muscle spasms or any of the other discomforts and agonies of the tank-bound. Many came to click from habit, involuntarily, even in their sleep. In dark wards at night, patients could be heard clicking, calling from their fitful sleep for help no one could give. Hospital workers once alert for the sound became inured to it, like city dwellers to the sound of sirens. I don't remember ever hearing my mother click, but I know she did. In 1992, when my first son was just a few months old, my grandmother and I were listening to him make the babbling baby sounds that precede speech when he discovered the giddyup-horse signal. My grandmother said softly, surprising me because she rarely spoke of my mother spontaneously, "That's the sound Virginia made when she needed help." After all those years, that simple, distinctive sound still held a power over my grandmother.

Sitting there with Maurine, who is forty-eight years older than I am, and my son, who is forty-one years younger, I thought of my absent mother and the children I didn't dare to have with my first husband—the children I wasn't brave enough to love and risk losing. Too much a child in need, then, myself. That day, with my own child in my arms, sitting beside my mother's mother, I became aware of a new loss: my mother as grandmother. She would not know my children, just as she had not known hers; they would not have her love and care, as we had not. Jens Husted, the man I married not long after my return to Colorado, and I now have two sons, and our boys have no grandmothers. Jens's mother died in 1954, just months after my mother became ill, in the sudden and spectacular way that bulbar polio can kill, leaving behind her husband and four children, ages two, four (Jens), six, and eight. For Jens and me, the loss of our mothers is not merely a coincidence, but a significant link. When we first began to talk of our losses, a few years ago, we discovered a shared, arcane language, one we had never spoken with anyone before.

AT SOME TIME during Mother's first, drifting weeks of illness, my grandparents returned to their home in Boulder, where Hayes went back to his job at the post office and my grandmother to her housewifery. There they waited and marked their days. Fred Davis wrote of the shock that polio brought to families. To see a family member healthy and active one day and "to be forced, a day or so later, to consider the likelihood of his dying, being crippled, or compelled to live in a mechanical respirator entails a most dramatic and disruptive alteration in fundamental perspectives." During this crisis, he wrote, "time is stripped of its familiar contexts as new and disturbing events quickly succeed and overlap each other."

No one in my family remembers exactly when, but sometime that summer the company Dad worked for gave him and a friend time off to drive Kenny and me to Colorado. We had not once been to the hospital to see Mother. We knew nothing of what had become of her since the June morning she and Dad had left to visit the doctor. She was simply gone. I can hardly bear to contemplate the heartbreak that I, as a four-year-old, suffered at my mother's disappearance. Mother was the one whose constant touch and voice and care I depended on and reveled in daily. And then, inexplicably, she was gone. I doubt I found much comfort in being told that she missed me, too, if anyone said that. But I do know I thought I had done something to send her away. I know I stood naked, vulnerable, and afraid without her protection. I know because I was to go on thinking and feeling that way for the next thirty years. My mother's sudden disappearance showed me that even the formless threat a child dreads most—the loss of a parent—can come to pass. The knowledge that the worst of disasters can strike the heart of my home is something I've carried with me, like a heavy stone, ever since.

Dad drove us children in his '49 Dodge pickup away from Arizona where Mother lay in the hospital. We bounced along next to him in the big cab, looking out the split windshield past the cartoonish nose of the truck to the highway. Sometimes, sitting on our knees, resting our chins on the seat back, we peered out the tiny rear window at our household belongings jostling in the truck's stubby bed behind. Dad's work friend, Jim May, drove our family car, a two-door '49 Chevrolet weighted with yet more possessions.

The trip went smoothly until it came time for the Dodge to haul us over the Rocky Mountains. The fuel pump gave out and left us sitting by the side of the road in the heat to consider our options. A trucker stopped to help, perhaps taken by the sight of my brother and me, with our wide eyes and skinny legs, in the care of two men. With a heavy chain he hitched our pickup to his tractor trailer and pulled us over the crest of the Rockies, and we rolled on into Boulder. Dad left the pickup, his children, and boxes of belongings there. Then he and Jim drove back to Phoenix in the Chevy. Their onerous errand completed, the men resumed their jobs.

Dad went home to our Duppa Villa apartment, now empty of wife and children and most all else. I suspect he drank each night. I don't know when he had begun drinking, maybe during his Marine service, but there can be little doubt that that summer encouraged his journey toward alcoholism. He has been able to tell me little of what went on that summer, except to say that he prayed each night, to a God he had no confidence in, for his death or Mother's.

Each evening Dad visited Mother after work, and each evening when he left her, the two were engulfed by their solitary nightmares, Dad alone in our apartment, Mother in her metal skin. What prayerful petitions entered her mind, I don't know. Surely, though, when she was able, she prayed for an end to her misery, took inventory through the length of her body, testing each muscle, willing something to move, disbelieving what fate had dealt her, and believing change would come. And whether I was pedaling our rusty tricycle in the Duppa Villa courtyard, being towed over mountain passes, or lying on the bunk bed in my grandparents' basement, all I wanted, all I prayed for, was my mother's presence.

ONE DAY, WHEN MY GRANDPARENTS were still in Phoenix, a nurse asked my grandmother whether her daughter had always been so quiet. No, Maurine replied. Virginia had a strong mind and will and was known to speak them, even in disagreement with her mother. At first, talking had been almost impossible for Mother, with air escaping the hole in her throat, but as the bulbar polio retreated, she slowly began to swallow again, and to speak haltingly in an unfamiliar voice. She expelled words when the iron respirator forced air out of her lungs and fell silent when it cut her off to draw air in. To avoid choking, she learned not to swallow while the machine inhaled. Mostly she lay silent, noncommittal and unemotional, until one day she broke into uncontrollable weeping. But even that breakdown was impotent. Her screams were hoarse squeals, not the powerful bellows that could have expressed and released suffering. Her circumstances warranted fist pounding, flailing, kicking, something to spend the agony, but the disease rendered her all but powerless even to demonstrate grief.

Unrelenting in its cruelty, polio robbed many of its victims of the one thing that could have given them at least temporary escape: a deep sleep. Encased in iron lungs, tortured victims vainly chased slumber through long, fitful nights. They seldom were given sleeping medication for fear it would push them too far from consciousness. In the night, patients lay listening to the liquid noises of other inmates, the squish of rubber-soled nurses retreating in the corridor, and the rattle of orderlies pushing IV stands through an empty hall. When sleep eventually came, it stayed two, perhaps three hours. The desire of muscles yearning to stretch and shift compounded the physical pain; the mind with no peaceful resting place tortured itself with its own desires. Patients as severely affected as my mother must have felt that only their brains and hearts lived.

Arnold Beisser found that in an iron lung time changed: "Without motion, time seemed to have slowed so considerably that it almost stopped. . . . Without familiar sources of pleasure and meaning, there was no future. . . . The movement of time was blocked, making the present interminable, lifeless, and dead." He asked a nurse what time it was, then waited and waited before asking again, only to find that three minutes had passed.

Without time passing in a familiar manner, the severely ill lose the story line of their lives. The physician Howard Brody wrote: "The notions of personal responsibility and personal identity [make] sense only within . . . a narrative framework. Without the passage of time there can be no narration; events cannot take on the meaning that narrative gives them if they cannot be located in time. . . . If one's time sense is seriously distorted by sickness, then sickness threatens self-respect in this very basic fashion." Iron lung patients, including Mother, were suspended in the moment, the nearly unbearable present, and lost touch with external reality.

One young woman, a quadriplegic, lay awake night after night in her iron lung seeing "horribly mangled bodies" in the shadows on the ceiling. "Gruesome, indescribable hallucinations lurked at the edge of my consciousness, ready to pounce the moment I let down the barrier of poems and Bible passages I repeated through the hours I tried to force myself into blessed sleep," she said. One night she heard an ambulance approach the hospital and mistook it for a fire engine. Her imagination took hold of the idea and terrorized her at the thought of the hospital catching fire. How could the iron-lung patients be moved from the burning building with no electricity to the elevators, no live plugs to attach to? In her agony, she tried to imagine what would be worse—suffocating or burning. "I could feel the metal of my respirator getting hotter and hotter," she said, "an oven in which I was roasting to death."

The possibility that my mother suffered such imagined agonies sears me, and I want to think, because no one can ever tell me differently, that her mind was more peaceful during those weeks of physical torment and confinement. But I know that even if such speculation and hallucinations didn't torture her at night, then the very real problems that faced her must have: thoughts of what would become of my brother and me if she died, knowledge of the distress her illness caused her parents and husband and others who loved her. Perhaps more mundane thoughts went through her mind. A friend to a woman who had a case as severe as my mother's told me that the woman, who came down with polio in December, worried about whether the gifts she had bought and wrapped for her husband's business associates and employees were contaminated. "She never asked because she did not want to know if they all had to be burned. That was what she worried about when she was expected to die," her friend wrote to me. "She said she had to worry about something . . . other than herself." I wonder whether Mother was dismayed to think she might have unknowingly infected others, especially Kenny or me, and watched to see whether we would join her in the hospital ward.

FOR MOST OF MY LIFE, I saw the events that happened to our family from the point of view of the young girl I was then. Even in my mid-thirties when I began to try to uncover the mysteries of my family's past and to learn who my mother was, I still saw it all from the wounded girl's eyes. But when I became a mother myself, first at forty-one and then again less than two years later, my point of view shifted radically. Being responsible for my sons turned me into an adult as had nothing else in the forty years before. Now a mother, I began to identify with my own mother, woman-to-woman, and even to feel maternal toward her, and that brought a new torrent of sorrows. I now imagine how, in addition to all the miseries that enmeshed Mother in the hospital, the simple, raw loss of being away from her children would have hurt her. I identify with the leaden fear she must have felt in imagining Kenny or me in her condition and how her inability to care for us would have made her helplessness even more wretched. At some time in those first weeks Mother must have added to the initial anguish of "I'm in pain and I'm afraid" the thought "My children need me and I can't care for them"—a wholly different source of agony.

One of the few stories my grandmother told me about my mother's illness when I was growing up was that Mother had said, "I'm glad it was me instead of one of the kids." I now assume Maurine told me that to try to convey my mother's caring for us children. During those growing-up years, however, the story stirred guilt and shame. I heard in it "Maybe it *should* have been one of you kids." The implications of love were too subtle for my understanding. I needed something direct. Dependent as I was then on the goodwill of my grandmother, who never whispered words of affection in my ear at night, I suppose I wanted to hear her say that *she* was glad it wasn't one of her grandchildren. We're not given choices, of course, in who among those we love will be singled out for misery. But now as a mother, I feel certain my mother meant it when she said she would rather have had polio find her than her children. And I feel as unsure as ever that my grandmother, given the option, would have chosen a granddaughter over her daughter. I find comfort, however, in believing that if there was a glimmer of peace for Mother in her iron lung, it was knowing, as time passed, that her children were safe. Her future, however, and our family's remained unknown. Some patients did emerge from iron lungs and resume their normal lives, fully recovered. As for those who did not, it was too soon to contemplate the radically altered life that awaited them.

In his book *The Nature of Suffering*, the medical humanist Eric J. Cassell argued against the distinction physicians tend to draw between mind and body, saying that identifying suffering exclusively with bodily pain is "misleading and distorting, for it depersonalizes the sick patient," and is itself a source of suffering. "That bodily pain causes personal suffering," he wrote, "cannot . . . be understood until the dichotomy between mind and body is rejected." Writing long after polio had ceased to be a concern of American physicians, Cassell surely was not thinking of that disease when he argued his position, yet it's difficult to imagine an affliction more prone to imposing both mental and physical suffering on its victims.

According to Cassell, people in physical pain suffer most when "they feel out of control, when the pain is overwhelming, when the source of the pain is unknown, when the meaning of the pain is dire, or when the pain is apparently without end." In such situations, he wrote, people see pain as a threat to their existence—"not merely to their lives but their integrity as persons." I read this and have to admit that his description entirely fits Mother's condition in those first weeks. All the conditions that made physical pain greatest applied to her.

No one could tell Mother when her pain would end; no one could control it or infuse it with meaning, or even offer an explanation for what—beyond the word *polio*—was causing her pain. No answers could mitigate the suffering of victims as encompassed by the poliovirus as she was in the acute stages of illness.

The task of keeping her alive, especially that summer she lay entombed in Phoenix Memorial Hospital, was so great that even had her doctors been aware of the sophisticated notions Cassell holds, they would not have had time or opportunity to aid her, so busy would they have been with her time-consuming care. Fully conscious once her early fevered delirium had passed, which must have been a couple of weeks, she was left to her own depleted resources to fight her nightly demons.

Some polio patients at Phoenix Memorial shared rooms off the main corridor, but Mother and other iron-lung victims stayed in a large open room where staff could more easily tend them. Hospitals often grouped iron lungs in the open space around the nurses' station or even in view in the hallways. During the epidemic year of 1952, polio patients congested Phoenix Memorial, as they did so many other hospitals. But in the summer of 1954, though the hospital had available dozens of iron lungs, few were occupied. By July 1954, Arizona had forty-two cases, fewer than in the previous summer, but as the polio season progressed, more and more victims joined Mother. One weekend in mid-July seven new patients were admitted, bringing the hospital total to twenty-nine. Mother and a twelve-year-old boy were then the only ones in iron lungs. Within the week, another twelve-year-old boy, stricken with spinal and bulbar polio while playing a baseball game, joined them. He battled through the night, spared by a tracheotomy. With his neck swathed in a bandage over the new wound and a tube running to an oxygen tank, he survived and watched more children come: a nine-year-old girl, a four-week-old boy flown from Flagstaff, Arizona, then a ten-year-old boy, and later, brothers eight and ten years old from the southern part of the state. How haunting it must have been for Mother to be surrounded by the small, sober faces of suffering children, crying in the night for their own mothers.

In late August, three months into her stay, an eighteen-year-old Phoenix girl was admitted with bulbar polio. The others watched her in her wretchedness, gasping for each breath for almost two weeks, only to see her die. Polio patients in acute wards were seldom shielded from the deaths of others. Death was too common and hospitals too crowded to keep the fates of patients private. A woman hospitalized on Long Island, New York, in 1949, said that each day when she woke, someone would be gone, often a child. Thomas Karwaki was a sixteen-year-old boy when confined to a semiprivate room at the children's hospital during Buffalo's epidemic of 1944. At first he was an almost solitary patient there, but then the one or two new admissions a day became twenty a day, most of them children under twelve, "and the dying began." His room became a "way station" for death. He knew that when sheets were draped between him and the next patient, the person was soon to go. For those in iron lungs, the death signal was the passing of a nurse down the row of tanks, turning each mirror so the patients couldn't watch while a body was wheeled out in a now silent machine.

Ill in the epidemic of 1955, Louis Sternburg remembers the iron lung ward as a scene from a "medieval pest house, complete with the stink. We were helpless, and it was impossible to keep us clean all the time." At one time sixty iron lungs, one holding Sternburg, were placed together in Massachusetts General Hospital "in a chaos of machinery, cables, thunderous bellows, extra lungs out in the corridor, nurses scurrying about, anxious families, visitors tripping over the cables, doctors dealing with crisis after crisis of choking, seizures, heart failure." The atmosphere at Phoenix Memorial Hospital in the summer of 1954 was considerably calmer, but Mother's predicament was no less dangerous.

As THE MONTHS WORE ON with Mother submerged in hospital life, the break in our family deepened. Kenny and I, confused and lonely, limped through the summer in the care of our grandparents. Even families not separated by as much geographic distance as ours suffered at least temporary ruptures. The initial break came when loved ones were put into hospital isolation, often in unfamiliar or distant facilities, because only certain hospitals took care of polio patients. When New Yorker Joseph Boettjer's young daughter, Joanne, was diagnosed with polio, he took her into the backyard to take her photograph before driving her to the hospital. "Who knew what condition she would be in upon her return?" he wrote to me recently. "I can recall the look of fear and confusion on her face—and the look of anguish on my wife's." Once he and his wife admitted Joanne to the hospital, they weren't allowed to see her. Reluctant to leave, they drove around the grounds to the area where they thought she had been taken. "As we sat quietly for a moment in the back of the building we heard a child cry out several times, 'I want my Mommy.' We were almost certain it was Joanne. What a heart-wrenching scene! We would have been far better off not to have gone there." Another mother recalled taking her seven-year-old daughter to a children's hospital and being told "to go to the back door and a special hallway" and then "to go away." She was told not to try to see her daughter, though she could call the doctor each morning for news.

Hearing such stories of other children and knowing how my brother and I were wrenched from our mother stirs a callow anger in me that understanding will not temper. I know that several factors came together in the forties and fifties that bred and encouraged the separations that seem inhumane to me. Such policies were born of fear of polio's contagion, of strict rules about hospital visits, of desires to protect children, and of a failure to understand the needs of children. But how is it that my father and grandparents—and other adults—couldn't see that we children needed above all else to be with our mother? And if that wasn't possible, then that we needed whatever contact was possible—a photograph or visits to the hospital exterior. I know my father and grandparents were suffering their own immeasurable misery and that they were ill equipped by their own upbringings to deal with difficult emotions. But still, I wish I had had even a glimpse of the hospital where Mother had been taken.

Karen McGinnis, whose mother was similarly affected by polio as mine, told me of her mother's stay in an Indiana hospital an hour's drive from the McGinnis home. Every night after closing his grocery store, her father drove there to visit his wife and often took Karen and her two brothers. He parked the car as close to their mother's window as possible, then left the children with one of their aunts while he went in for a visit. "I remember once when it was light outside," Karen told me, "we were all standing on the ground looking up towards my mother's window and my father kept saying, 'There's your mother's room,' and telling us to wave and I couldn't understand why she would not come to the window and wave back. I wondered if she was standing there and I couldn't see her because of the bright glare of the sun. I remember standing there and waving and smiling but not being able to see her." Karen, like me, was four in 1954 when her mother went into an iron lung, and the image of her and her brothers waving at the empty window makes my heart ache—and yet I'm envious. As confused and lonely as I know those children were without their mother, at least they had a window, a place where they knew their mother was. My mother had simply vanished.

THE PAIN OF CHILDREN separated from their ill parents and of parents unable to comfort their sick children, considerable though it was, couldn't be matched by the anxiety and isolation of the children left in hospitals. Sharon Stern came down with polio in 1954 when she was nine, and the night she was admitted to a New York hospital remains vivid in her memory. Already losing muscle strength, she was propped to a sitting position on an examination table. "I saw my reflection in the window. I remember looking past [it] through the windows of another wing of the hospital where I saw people moving about. I wondered if there was another child in all those windows or all the world who felt as miserable as I did. I wondered if anyone could know how utterly wretched I felt."

Each hospital that took patients with contagious diseases established quarantine periods. With polio, the length varied, sometimes widely because no one knew for certain how long patients were contagious, though most hospitals set ten days to three weeks as the isolation time. Dressed in white pajamas with big red dots on their backs to warn of contagion, children lay on beds and in oversized cribs beneath signs saying Polio. They had nothing to do, and they were in the company of strangers for the length of the isolation period. Some doctors didn't even enter the rooms of children with polio, but stood in the doorway or waved through a glass partition. When hospital staff did enter the children's rooms, they came covered in gowns and caps that they shed when they left. Doctors seldom touched the children, and when they did, it was with gloved hands. That separation caused pain to physicians as well, as Thomas Whitfield, the pediatrician who worked at Massachusetts General in the fifties, remembers: "You wanted to pick them up and hold them, and you just didn't do that."

Doris Seligman, a teenager in 1949 at Willard Parker Hospital in New York, lay "encased in an iron lung and isolated except for some rare contact with nurses . . . soaked in urine most of the time." She had so little attention that it was not until the night the hospital lost electrical power and someone rushed to hand pump her iron lung that she realized she wasn't forgotten. Some families of polio victims mounted twenty-four-hour bedside vigils. For months, Ohioan Jack Clements, whose twenty-one-year-old wife, Bette, was fully paralyzed in 1955, kept round-the-clock watch over her, taking shifts with the aunt and uncle who had reared her. For the first couple of months she couldn't even speak, and they feared leaving her alone. They developed a code of eye blinks and lip reading to communicate with her. The company Jack worked for gave him a fully paid leave, and he sat in a wheelchair at her head from 7:00 P.M. until noon the next day. When she could again speak, he went back to work, but still spent his nights there from 9:00 P.M. until he went to work in the morning.

Many hospitals, however, kept family members away in the first days or even weeks. Parents desperate for glimpses of their stricken children held in isolation leaned ladders against hospital walls and climbed to peer in the windows. One mother sneaked into a hospital contagious ward, hoping to see her child, and was quarantined herself when hospital personnel discovered her. In New York, a young woman still in isolation looked up in surprise, then dread, to see her mother standing at her bedside. "How did you get in here?" she asked. "Oh, you know me," her mother said, "I just wormed my way in." But the daughter knew that her mother's cheerfulness was a shield for what every patient on the floor knew: Visitors were allowed only when doctors thought the patient wouldn't live much longer.

Other mothers stayed away, fearing they would bring polio home to their healthy children. In 1944, one seven-year-old boy in Buffalo who couldn't breathe declined steadily over three days and died without seeing his mother, who lived just a few blocks away. In the months Mother lay in the Phoenix hospital, with not a single glimpse of her children, she must have known that we'd been taken to Colorado and that no emergency would bring us back to her. She must have realized that she could die any moment without the chance to kiss us goodbye. At the time, we all thought her condition was a nightmare that would end. But now, I look back and see that her time in the Arizona hospital, with our family splintered, was the beginning of the end for us. I see now that the devastating crevasse begun then would become unbreachable.

The gowns, masks, caps, gloves, and bowls of soapy disinfectant in the halls, and the long hours and days alone, distanced polio patients of all ages from their families and the rest of their community. But youngsters, lacking understanding of their situation, suffered in their own particular, grievous way. Six-year-old David Heming, in isolation at a hospital in Moose Jaw, Saskatchewan, for nine weeks saw his parents only from his fifth-floor window. They came faithfully each day for the little contact with him they could have. "I could not understand why they put me in the hospital," he remembered years later. "Why they put me away like this. I could not understand why they didn't come and take me home." One day they left a bouquet of sweet peas from their garden, which the nurses took to him in his ward. Decades later, the scent of sweet peas still made him gag.

Some hospitals allowed families to visit contagious wards, but the rule was "look, don't touch." Parents pressed against windows dividing the hale from the ill for views of their children. They talked to loved ones through the transom over the door or at the threshold to a room they were forbidden to enter. But they didn't always obey the regulations; when no one was looking, parents crept across the room to kiss their paralyzed children and touch their feverish faces.

Once patients served their isolation periods and moved to regular wards, hospital rules often continued to keep them apart from family members, not because they had polio, but simply because that's how hospitals operated then. The liberal visiting hours at most of today's hospitals were unheard of then. Visiting might be restricted to specific weekend hours only, or from 7:00 P.M. to 7:30 P.M. daily, and children were seldom allowed into hospitals at all.

I've seen photographs of people in iron lungs with mementos taped to the tanks over their heads, keeping them company through the absences from family, and I've wondered whether Mother had any pictures of our family in her view. Trying to imagine what snapshots might have been there, I pulled out the few from our family's Arizona days, all of them from those weekend outings to the desert. I stare at them and see her beautiful body, her long, slender neck and arms. In one photograph she's squatting, wearing a strapless polka-dot bra-top and shorts. She's as tan as a fair-skinned woman can possibly be and has an arm wrapped around each of us children. We are as brown as she. In one hand she holds a cigarette, a touch I find slightly glamorous and grown-up in the way it was in the fifties. In another photo she is standing in front of a giant saguaro cactus and squinting into the sun, with one hand resting casually on Kenny's shoulder, the other on mine. We're leaning into her. I wonder whether from her iron lung she could have looked at our grins and bare feet without her heart breaking any more than I can look at them today.

HOSPITAL VISITS SHAPED THE LIVES of both patients and families. Sharon Stern's mother came to see her in her iron lung during the daytime visiting hours, and her father came for the evening visits. Orthodox Jews, they didn't drive on the Sabbath, so her father took the car to the hospital late Friday afternoons, visited Sharon, and walked home. On Saturday evenings her parents walked to the hospital, visited Sharon, and then drove the car home. For many hospitalized patients, the regular visits, which sometimes came only weekly, became the one island of respite in their hospital days.

Often the weeks of isolation progressed to weeks on a general ward, then to more weeks of rehabilitation. The world of polio victims shrank to their rooms and wards; as for those in iron lungs, they lost contact with everything beyond the metal shell in which they lived. I don't know whether any news of the world outside the hospital penetrated to Mother during that long summer in Phoenix. Joseph McCarthy, the Senate's headhunter of Communists, drew headlines with his search through the U.S. Army for Red sympathizers, and a record-breaking heat wave killed people across the country; but such events would have seemed strangely remote to a person fighting for life. I wonder, though, whether anyone told Mother of the sudden death of twenty-year-old Emilie Dionne, one of the famous Dionne quintuplets, who died that August of a stroke. Five thousand people gathered for her funeral at the Dionne home in Ontario. The young woman and her four sisters had been a source of fascination not only for my mother, who was eight when they were born, but for countless others worldwide. With the help of her aunt Lourie, Mother, as a child, had kept a scrapbook of newspaper clippings about the quints, following the five girls as they, and Mother, grew up. Back in Boulder, Lourie clipped the front-page stories chronicling the world's grief at the loss and recapturing the unusual story of the Dionne sisters. She saved the stories, adding them to the others, and must have hoped to show them to Mother when she was well and home again. I don't know whether Mother ever saw them, but I did, once, as a girl, when Aunt Lourie, who still lived next door to my grandparents, showed the scrapbook to me.

The confinement of one family member always causes disruptions in family life, but when a parent becomes ill, families suffer special stresses. Fred Davis reported in *Passage through Crisis: Polio Victims and Their Families* that when, as in our family, an adult fell seriously ill, "many of the . . . central functions of family life—breadwinning, child care, housekeeping, sex, recreation—" were vitally disrupted. The effects were so pronounced that the family found it exceedingly difficult "to reconstruct the experience so that it 'fit in,' psychologically speaking, with a known past and an imagined future."

Caught as our family was on the brink of a move, we experienced an extreme disruption, individually and as a group. We weren't rooted in a home or community, and we didn't have a life that could go on around the same kitchen table while we waited for Mother's return. When she fell ill, everything about our life changed, rocking our family identity.

ARNOLD BEISSER, RENDERED QUADRIPLEGIC and unable to breathe by polio, much later wrote that, separated as he was in his iron lung from the elemental functions and activities that occupy people—even breathing—his "place in the culture was gone." Mother lost her personal identity as well, at least for a time, because nothing intensified the isolation of polio patients as much as the iron lung. My mother, a woman of twenty-eight, accustomed to the embraces of two eager children and a young husband, was now touched only when gloved hospital staff needed to tend her body: wipe it clean, draw blood, feed it, shift its position. Unable to move, she could no longer perform any of the small or grand routines and activities of her life. Beisser wrote: "At times I felt as if I had lost my human qualities, and did not belong to the species *Homo sapiens* any longer. . . . I had become a 'thing.' I had no words that could adequately describe what

I felt. I was exposed utterly and completely. I was vulnerable to everyone and everything. Nothing was private; there was only wordless shame for what I had become. Logic and rationality were useless to me." Each time I read those words, I'm struck by the torment Mother experienced, and I mourn, especially over the "wordless shame."

To Beisser, only his head seemed familiar, protruding from one end of the tank as "the only part that remained recognizably human." In his iron lung, his body no longer belonged to him. "Entry beneath my new metal skin was at the discretion of others. Those who attended to my body did things when and how they believed they should be done, and I seemed to have little or no part in this. . . . My head was treated as if it was separated from the rest of my body. People exchanged views with it as an equal, and they even asked permission before doing things to it."

The iron respirators, those life-saving prisons, revolutionized the treatment of the most serious forms of polio. Until the thirties, doctors could do almost nothing for patients suffering paralysis of the breathing muscles. They could only watch as the first signs of respiratory distress came on, knowing their patient might live a few more hours, a damned day or two at most. Manual methods could keep a patient breathing for a short time, but every type of resuscitation known proved exhausting to both the victim and the rescuers and could not be sustained for any length of time.

Since the 1830s, various inventors, even Alexander Graham Bell, had tinkered with devising some kind of external respiration. Then in the fall of 1926, chemical engineer Philip Drinker of the Harvard School of Public Health happened upon a breathing machine that radically changed the care of polio patients. Watching a colleague use a machine to measure the breathing of an animal, he got the idea for a tank respirator. He had a local tinsmith build a human-sized box, and added to it a salvaged pair of used vacuum-cleaner blowers and the necessary valves. He then sealed an end plate with a rubber collar to the device. Over two years Drinker and his colleagues worked on the design, trying to create a machine that provided adequate ventilation. Drinker himself was one of the first human subjects to test it.

Then on October 12, 1928, an eight-year-old girl was admitted to Children's Hospital of Boston with fever, headache, stiffness of neck and back, weakness of the left arm, and some respiratory difficulty. A spinal fluid analysis told doctors she had polio, and her persistent fever warned that the damage could be extensive. Drinker's apparatus stood ready. A day later the hospital called Drinker to come quickly. He found the girl dangerously blue, unconscious in the silent machine. The staff had been afraid to turn on the power. He started the pump, and in a few minutes the girl's normal color returned and she regained consciousness. She tried to speak, but didn't know how to coordinate her words with the pressure of the machine. Once she got the hang of it, she asked for ice cream, and thus brought tears to the eyes of those who witnessed the scene, including Drinker.

Over the next days they moved her in and out of the tank—out to breathe with her still-functioning diaphragm, in to rest. They found she could clear her throat and cough in the machine, which had been difficult outside. They found she could also eat and sleep there. When pneumonia developed, she wanted to be in the tank more. Writing for the *Journal of the American Medical Association* in 1929 about his new apparatus, Drinker said: "In her own words, she could 'breathe bigger' in the tank than outside it. If the negative pressure fell . . . , she generally asked us to 'run it more.' " James L. Wilson, who as a hospital resident helped care for that girl, wrote in his memoirs: "One could hear it running for a quarter of a mile away because it was summer and the windows were all open. All of the residents, including myself, took turns sitting up with this child day and night." Despite such care, she died on October 19 though until the last minutes her color stayed good and she remained conscious and alert. Although the child died, apparently from cardiac failure, the principle of external ventilation had been established.

In 1929 just one respirator, which cost two thousand dollars to build, existed in the world. But as word of the device spread, the machines could not be made fast enough. Drinker answered phone calls at all hours from around the world, giving instructions on how to build and operate them.

Officially the machine was known as the Drinker respirator or Drinker lung, though when a journalist dubbed it the "iron lung," a name all too suitable, that stuck. People also called it the Emerson tank, after the primary manufacturer, J. H. Emerson Company in

Cambridge. At least one baby boy was named Emerson by his grateful mother who, while pregnant, had been saved by the mechanical breather.

A severe epidemic in 1931 put the tanks in great demand, but few hospitals had enough lungs to accommodate patients, making for agonizing decisions. People died for lack of an iron lung; others died when weaned too early in an effort to make the machine available to someone in greater distress. The hope was that the machines would, as Drinker wrote in 1929, "give all patients with respiratory paralysis [the] opportunity to recover normal breathing by maintaining artificial respiration over a period of hours, or even days." What happened, however, was that some patients stayed not hours or days in the metal sheaths, but months, even years.

In the thirties, nurses and doctors trained in their use were as limited as the tanks. When the physician John Paul, who was with the Yale Poliomyelitis Unit, went into a rural area to study an epidemic, he spent most of his time "as a not-too-well-trained supervisor directing nurses in the use of the respirator." Once the National Foundation for Infantile Paralysis formed, however, in the late 1930s, it took up the cause of trying to supply hospitals in epidemic areas with both equipment and trained staff. The Los Angeles County Hospital in 1948 cared for 2,900 polio cases, nearly one-tenth of all the cases in the United States—and 280 of those patients needed iron lungs. Army airplanes flew respirators to the city, and at one time 82 pumped in that one hospital alone. When an epidemic hit Massachusetts in 1955, the NFIP rushed 204 iron lungs from all parts of the country to that state. In Michigan's Upper Peninsula a mechanically minded resident built an iron lung himself to have one on hand, should anyone in the area need it, according to Donald Thurber, who became the Michigan director of the NFIP in 1943. The man, he recalled, "was hailed as a kind of local hero."

The iron lung became an icon of the polio years. At the 1933–34 Chicago World's Fair crowds lined up in the Hall of Science to see it. In the "Dick Tracy" comic strip, Tracy once rushed a child to an iron lung. Newspaper cartoonists showed it resuscitating defeated politicians, as well as the deflated currency of 1933.

WHEN MOTHER NEEDED AN IRON LUNG at the beginning of the 1954 polio season, several stood empty at Phoenix Memorial, thoroughly checked by mechanics, ready for the need that would no doubt come as the summer progressed. Hospitals equipped to care for polio victims sometimes employed engineers around the clock to keep the respirators operating. Once in use, the machines, which used about as much electrical current as a household refrigerator, often had to run six months without stopping. In the case of mechanical or electrical failure, an alarm on top of the respirator sounded, and built-in, hand-operated bellows kept the patient breathing.

From the beginning of my search into my family's past, I was both repelled and fascinated by the iron lung. The researcher in me decided it would be interesting to take a close look at one, maybe even climb in and let it breathe for me. I figured that with a few telephone calls I could find one. As reasonable as that sounds, however, I found I couldn't go through with it. In my imagination and nightmares I have done time in an iron lung. I've been in one alone and with my mother. I've heard its maddening din. I've seen Mother's face on the head of every iron lung patient I've looked at in photographs. I've struggled to breathe and be free of the tank, and I simply cannot voluntarily, physically climb into one.

NOT EVERYONE INSIDE AN IRON LUNG was as immobile as my mother. Because of the individual way in which polio struck, some patients couldn't breathe, but could move their legs and arms. Some had paralyzed trunk muscles, but able limbs. One woman couldn't lift her shoulders or upper arms from the bed, but could move her arms to the side of the lung and back by crawling with her fingers. Nurses gathered around to cheer when a patient discovered a new movement—a flexed finger, a foot that wiggled, or toes that curled. Every motion was hailed, wisely or not, as a step toward recovery.

Unable to move or breathe, iron-lung patients watched visitors and hospital workers moving and breathing. Stagnant, they waited for something to happen. If placed near a window, they could watch the street, giving them something to look at, something to think about as a change from long hours of staring at the ceiling or into a mirror above their heads that reflected reversed, distorted images from the hospital room. In the fifties, some fortunate few who had televisions in their wards watched baseball players run from third to first base in a left-hand world. Others listened to programs on rented radios. Special devices projected book pages onto the ceiling, and a sensitive electronic control resting against the patient's cheek turned pages when the command was given by the pressure of the tongue. But most patients who read did so with books placed on overhead racks, and they waited for someone to come along to turn pages. I heard of a woman who read three books at a time, choosing ones different in tone and subject so she could keep them straight in her mind, because that gave her six pages to read at once and lengthened the time her page-turner could be away doing something else.

I wonder whether Mother had any interests that could have occupied her during those months in the Phoenix hospital or whether she was so ill she couldn't even read. I try to imagine what would have brought her pleasure and find again how little I know about her. I have just one book that was hers, the 1939 "Illustrated Motion Picture Edition" of *Gone with the Wind*, a large paperback with color photographs from the movie. I don't know whether the book reflected her literary tastes or merely the popularity of the book and movie.

ALTHOUGH PHOENIX MEMORIAL had the facilities and staff for rehabilitation and did teach many patients skills they needed once they went home, its main job was to care for acute polio patients. Respiratory patients whose conditions stabilized but who would need long-term care or rehabilitation, like my mother, were transferred to other treatment centers. After almost four months flat on her back in her iron lung at Phoenix Memorial, Mother was told she would be moved to a place where she could be evaluated and treated by respiratory specialists.

The nearest center for the rehabilitation of respiratory patients, Rancho Los Amigos Medical Center in California, was full.

She would go, instead, to the new Northwest Respirator Center in Seattle.

Moving patients in iron lungs even within a hospital was laborious and potentially dangerous. Moving them across town required wiring elevators and hallways, and having ready a van or truck that could haul the six-hundred-pound machine and that was loaded with a gasoline generator to keep the lung pumping during transport. A forklift, a back-up generator, oxygen supplies, and a nurse and doctor were good to have along, too. In some cities, such moves to other hospitals or rehabilitation centers were made with the help of the U.S. Army and local fire departments. Some patients moving longer distances went by train, as did a twenty-year-old man who was transferred from a California hospital to the Seattle center. He rode in a baggage car outfitted by Southern Pacific Railroad and was accompanied by a doctor, two nurses, and an electrician.

Others, like my mother, traveled by airplane, ideally, a C-47 Skytrain, the workhorse of both civilian airlines and of the Allied war effort during World War II and the Korean War. The twin-engine propeller plane proved valuable in flying polio patients, not only because it was reliable, durable, and widely available, but also because it had a door wide enough to push an iron lung through. Small, portable lungs made especially for transportation were rare, so most people flew in conventional-sized lungs. Too confining for daily use, the portables were never made in great numbers.

As with many transfers of polio patients, Mother's was arranged and paid for by the state NFIP office, which enlisted the help of the Military Air Transport Service (MATS). Beginning in 1950, MATS, a part of the U.S. Air Force that airlifted passengers, troops, and tons of cargo daily, was enlisted to help fly polio patients to treatment hospitals and polio equipment to epidemic areas. In January 1953 the NFIP presented MATS a citation of honor to recognize the service's efforts.

On Monday morning, September 27, 1954, Mother was unplugged from Phoenix Memorial Hospital, attached to a generator, and driven, still in her iron lung, to Luke Air Field, where Lieutenant Colonel George M. Sabin Jr. and a crew of four others from Luke waited. For some reason the nurse and doctor from Phoenix Memorial who often accompanied patients on transfer flights did not go with Mother. Instead, someone from the NFIP had called Luke Air Force Base saying they needed a physician to accompany her on her flight. When the call came in, Sabin, the physician who was the base hospital commander, could have assigned the job to any of the doctors under him, but decided to go himself. He and Mother were joined by a nurse, a nonmedical officer, the pilot, and the copilot on the fifteen-hundred-mile flight.

When Mother arrived at the airfield, television cameras followed her aboard the Douglas C-47 cargo plane. She was hoisted in her tank, along with a generator and suction machine and a tangle of cables, into the plane, resting on its three wheels, its bullet nose twenty feet off the ground.

Dad climbed on, too, to make sure the iron lung was fastened down securely, to kiss Mother goodbye, and to offer whatever reassurances were possible. He was not traveling with her, but would stay with his job a couple more months and then follow in the Chevy. He lingered a moment too long, and when he heard the revving of the engines, a sound familiar to the soldier in him who had flown night missions, he shouted to the crew, "I'm not going! I need to get off!" The television camera captured his sheepish grin as he scrambled from the Skytrain, giving a jaunty, cheerful air to the event. The television commentator, interpreting the handsome smile as strength in adversity, said of my ex-Marine father, "That's why we win wars." Dad's friends later told him he looked good on TV, but he missed the broadcast himself.

The airplane door closed on Mother and she flew, alone and helpless, accompanied by people she'd never seen before who would turn her over to the care of other strangers in a place she knew nothing of—a place farther from her Colorado home and her children and parents and the mountains she longed to see.

Forty years later when I found Sabin, now retired, to ask whether he remembered flying with my mother to Seattle, I learned he did, because it was the only such flight he'd made. Smooth and uneventful was how he remembered it. He gave me copies of letters from his files about the episode. One was sent the day after to the base commander, a brigadier general, from the state NFIP representative, who expressed her "deep appreciation" to the crew who "transported Mrs. Virginia Black, polio respirator patient" for their "magnificent job." The commander then sent a copy of it to Lieutenant Colonel Sabin, saying it gave him "great pleasure" to forward the attached letter. "The efficient manner in which this 'mercy flight' to Seattle, Washington was performed reflects favorably upon your professional abilities and the U.S. Air Force." He added: "Our accomplishment of missions such as this gives us an opportunity to tell the general public that the Air Force is not only prepared for war but is also eager to assist in peaceful endeavors."

Holding the carbon-smudged letters in my hands intensified an odd, but now familiar, detachment from my mother, created by the long years and those terrible events. Reading "Mrs. Virginia Black, polio respirator patient" on official stationery, seeing that the U.S. Air Force deemed something she was involved in as a "mercy flight" and cause for congratulations stirs no feeling. I struggle to find a point of reference in those words. Mrs. Virginia Black, polio respirator patient. I struggle to see in them a trace of Mother.

MOTHER'S TRANSFER SIGNALLED that she had passed through two important stages: she'd survived the initial onslaught of polio and had reached a stable existence in the iron lung. Now, perhaps, in this new place, something could change. I wonder whether, during the flight to Seattle, she believed she would one day walk onto an airplane there and fly, like an ordinary passenger, home to Colorado. Doctors in Phoenix had not offered predictions about her future. Did that mean anything was possible? Did that mean she might again touch her children, make love, cook dinner, dance? Whatever she believed might happen to her, she must have hoped this journey northwest would lead her eventually to Colorado, where Kenny and I and her parents kept loyal watch.

CHAPTER FOUR

Hot Packs, Exercise, and Prayer

The treatment and rehabilitation a patient received naturally depended on the type of polio and the extent of the paralysis. Many people recovered completely, or nearly so. Those left with residual paralysis faced a range of ill effects, from the minor to the life-changing. Like others beset by misfortune, polio patients found solace in comparing themselves to others. Taking note of those worse off was an attempt, as Fred Davis remarked in his study of families with children who had polio, to find "a symbolic resting place for themselves within some calculable scheme of human advantages and infirmities." Patients on crutches prayed for the day they could throw the sticks away, while patients who couldn't use their arms or legs left crutches at religious shrines and prayed to be able to use them one day. Hospitalized patients rated their polio woes. A man confined for months with polio as a boy remembered thinking: "Well, I'm stuck in bed here, but . . . at least I can turn the pages of this book with my finger and don't have to do it by using a stick in my mouth. I'm a lucky guy!" Patients at Warm Springs had a saying: "If you have to get polio, get it when you're five; if you have to get it, get it in the legs." Surely, if Warm Springs had had respiratory cases, the maxim would have gone on: "And whatever you do, don't get polio in your twenties and don't get it in your breathing muscles."

My mother was among the most devastated of polio victims. She was as ill, as paralyzed, as one could be and still be alive. Quadriplegics on respirators, like her, were at the end of the line, and little comfort for them could be found in comparisons.

THE TREATMENT AND REHABILITATION a patient received also depended, I learned, on circumstances. What kind of community the patient lived in (large or small, prepared for polio cases or not, close to a specialized treatment center or not) and how many other polio cases were around could profoundly affect the care a victim received. Being the single polio patient in a hospital, for instance, could mean you were the object of a great deal of attentive care from a medical staff that had plenty of time for you. Or it could mean being cared for by people who had no idea what to do for you, a little like depending on your internist to do heart surgery. Coming down with polio during an epidemic might mean you were cared for with the best of specialized medical workers and equipment, brought to your community by state agencies and the NFIP. Or it could mean you received no care at all.

In 1950, *Collier's* magazine sounded the alarm for local communities with an article titled "If Polio Strikes . . . Is Your Town Ready?" It compared 1949 epidemics in Maine and Arkansas, two states hit hard that year by polio. Maine, with a population of one million, had 463 polio cases and only 10 deaths. Arkansas, with twice the population and twice the number of cases, had five times as many deaths. The explanation, the reporter suggested, might lay in preparedness. Maine had in place a plan for medical mobilization and convalescent care. Three of the state's largest hospitals were prepared to accept acute polio patients when the polio season opened. In Arkansas, however, it was not until mid-July, when nearly three hundred cases of polio had been reported, that officials even recognized they had a serious epidemic on their hands. The entire state had but twelve iron lungs, and far too few hospital beds and trained nurses for their growing number of patients. With the help of the Red Cross and the NFIP, 252 beds, 36 respirators, and 184 nurses were rounded up from other states and freighted or flown into Arkansas. But despite these measures, by the end of the polio season, the state had been overwhelmed by their one thousand cases of polio.

This meant that some patients, like one two-year-old from a poor Arkansas farming family, received no care. When the girl fell ill, her parents took her to a local doctor, who immediately diagnosed polio and ordered her rushed in an ambulance to a hospital—not the nearest one, but the only one in the state that took polio patients, in Little Rock, 175 miles of rough road away. Clutching the hand of her worried and confused mother, the girl endured the painful six-hour ambulance journey, only to find bedlam at the end of the line. The hospital's thirty-bed isolation ward overflowed; patients lay on stretchers on the corridor floors, and panic-stricken parents swarmed the building. The isolation ward was already crowded with cases of other illnesses when the first five polio victims arrived in May. One hundred more polio patients soon followed. A room intended for a single patient held six beds. Four cribs were packed so tightly into a cubicle that nurses had to move three of them to attend to the fourth baby. In the midst of such chaos someone in a white coat examined the girl and then told her mother she'd be better off at home. The mother picked up the girl and carried her to the ambulance. Six hours later they were back where they had started.

That fall, a medical social worker paid for by the NFIP found the girl at her home. She had survived polio, but her right leg was weak and deformed, and her right arm dangled loosely. Weeks of visits from the social worker finally persuaded the mother to allow a doctor to take a look at her child. The girl's right arm was fitted with a brace, and exercises were prescribed for the leg, in hopes that it would strengthen with time. She never fully recovered.

Looking back now, there's no way to know how much of polio's residual crippling or even how many deaths could have been prevented with prompt diagnoses and the best of care available in the postwar decade. All we can say for certain is that care, both treatment and rehabilitation, varied widely and that many polio victims received less than the best.

Frances Billings Finke, who fell ill with a severe case in 1944, was one such patient. Fully paralyzed with her head twisted to the back, the teenager rode in an ambulance to a hospital in nearby La Crosse, Wisconsin, where she lay in an iron lung for five weeks without any physical therapy, stiffening like a corpse, her head still twisted painfully. In the sixth week she began breathing outside the lung and was transferred to another hospital, where hot packs and physical therapy began. She was so rigid that each joint had to be broken loose. Therapy went on, but no one ever applied hot packs to her hands. They did to her feet, feet she would never walk on again; but her gnarled hands, worked regularly and painfully in physical therapy, were never softened with hot packs. She always wondered whether better, more prompt care of her hands might have made a difference in the long run.

ALL THOSE WHO CONTRACTED POLIO in the postwar decade, if nothing else, could be thankful that they'd escaped the remedies of the past century. No treatment at all was surely better than the nine-teenth-century methods of bleeding (as was done for most any ail-ment). Doctors then also applied ice to the spines of polio patients or rubbed on mercury ointment to produce blisters; hoping to awaken paralyzed limbs, they jolted hapless patients with electrical current. One doctor in 1872 told his medical students that he favored applying a red-hot iron over the affected area until an ulcer formed. Another medical authority writing in 1911 advocated amputation of paralyzed limbs, heaping more trauma on the patient.

From the earliest times, treatment of polio patients was dis-couraging to physicians. This terrible disease that couldn't be pre-vented, couldn't be effectively treated either. "The best that could be said is that the physician of the nineteenth and early twentieth centu-ries," wrote John R. Paul, "generally had faith in his remedies—faith which he sometimes was able to instill into his patients." In the epi-demic of 1916, physicians could do little more for the thousands who fell ill than advise bed rest. As the years went on, the accepted regi-men became one of immobilizing the affected limbs, followed by massage and hydrotherapy, and much later, once deformities had set-tled in, surgery, if needed.

By the 1930s belief in the value of immobilizing limbs during the acute stage evolved into immediate and prolonged rigid splinting and casting of limbs. Encased in plaster, legs down, arms outstretched as if crucified, patients lay in convalescent hospitals. Some were placed in beds framed with ropes and pulleys to prevent movement. Occasionally, children with even mild cases were dressed in casts or splints to immobilize limbs. Doctors reasoned that limbs left untreated would draw into deformity by strong muscles pulling against weakened ones.

Until the forties, treatment of polio patients rested mainly in the hands of orthopedists, who found little reward in the task. All their efforts at casting and splinting left them legions of crippled and deformed children, yet all the doctors could offer were surgeries that not only were marginally effective but were beyond what most patients could afford.

By 1940, many in medicine had observed that the use of splints and casts had gone too far. "Incredibly, immobility had become such a fetish that it was proposed even as a preventive measure for 'keeping the paralysis away,' " wrote Paul. Prolonged fixation often lead to irreversible damage as muscles atrophied.

As if on cue, Elizabeth Kenny, a nurse from Australia, arrived in the United States in 1940 to challenge conventional thinking. Her experience in the Australian bush with paralytic polio had convinced her that doctors placed too much emphasis on prolonged rest at the expense of other, more helpful therapy. She called casts and splints illogical, said that holding paralyzed limbs immobile not only did no good but did harm, and set out to change the way American doctors cared for polio patients. "In retrospect," wrote Paul, "there is no denying that Sister Kenny's ideas and techniques marked a turning point, even an about-face, in the aftercare of paralytic poliomyelitis. By determination and sheer willpower she helped to raise the treatment of paralyzed patients out of the slough into which it had sunk in the 1930s."

The about-face came quickly, though not easily and not without controversy. By late 1942, an orthopedist on the NFIP advisory board said: "Continuous rigid splinting is not only on its way out, it is out." By 1947 the NFIP sold for scrap thousands of splints it had kept on hand for epidemics. One foundation official, on a visit to Warm Springs, saw that a farmer living near the rehabilitation center had used the splints in his garden as poles for beans.

To the public, Sister Kenny was the angel of mercy they had been waiting for. She told of bringing paralyzed children back "to normalcy" from paralytic polio—welcome news to Americans who felt helpless in the face of the advancing invader. Her title "Sister" was the British term for *nurse*, but to American ears, for whom the term conjured thoughts of nuns, Kenny had a saintly air.

MANY PHYSICIANS, HOWEVER, OPPOSED both Kenny and her ideas. Soon after her arrival in the United States, a reporter for the *American Weekly* magazine visited Minnesota General Hospital to observe her methods. He praised the "courageous" doctors who worked with her: "Why call physicians courageous simply because they permit Sister Kenny to demonstrate her method of polio aftercare? Simply because it seems very doubtful to the medical profession as a whole that a nurse who began her treatment in far-off Australia some 30 years ago—and in the hinterland where there was no doctor within 100 miles—could make a significant contribution to the knowledge about infantile paralysis." As many other magazine and newspaper reporters did, this writer related the "relief from distressing pain which is a symptom of the acute, early stages of this cruel disease" and the "remarkable recoveries from crippling deformities" that her methods brought. A photograph showed a little girl with a twisted hip and shortened leg after more than a year of conventional treatment. Next to it, another photo showed her after just three days of Kenny's treatment method: the distorted hip had straightened so that the legs were the same length.

Again and again the extraordinary nurse performed what the press liked to call "miracles," a term that never failed to annoy her. " 'All I did,' she would say, 'was straighten a pelvic obliquity, something I have done many times before.' " Which is just what she might have said about that little girl's hip in those magazine photos.

Scenes like one played out on November 12, 1943, before a group of forty doctors and a number of nurses and therapists at the cramped solarium atop Adelphi Hospital in Brooklyn drew public adulation. That day, she worked on an eight-year-old boy who had not moved his deformed left leg in two years. Examining the leg, she determined that he wasn't paralyzed but that the muscles were "alienated." That is, when he was sick, it hurt to move the leg, and so he didn't. Once the pain receded, his muscles had been still so long that they'd lost the notion of movement. Relax, she told him. Think of your foot, she said, as she moved the leg; now you try. He did, and the leg moved. More than a thousand doctors and parents telephoned the hospital following the reports of that demonstration and asked for treatment for children and various other patients. Still, many of her critics continued to explain her work as either a special gift of hers that couldn't be taught to others, or as "spontaneous recoveries." More and more, however, physicians who saw her work were won over.

Her life took on a romanticized glow when the 1946 Hollywood version of her story, called *Sister Kenny*, chronicled her Australian days and her move to the United States. Her story of a lone nurse struggling against powerful doctors, with the well-being of defenseless children at stake, was ripe for the movies. When *Sister Kenny* opened in New York at the RKO Palace, it drew twenty thousand people to Times Square and helped bond the public to her as their savior from the dread disease.

She projected an imposing physical presence, if not a saintly one. Tall, broad shouldered, and big bosomed, dressed in black or navy blue, she emphasized her size with large hats and giant flowers pinned to her chest. Her face wasn't in the least like that of Rosalind Russell, who played her in the movie. In fact, Carolee Cornelius Burris, who as a girl was a patient of hers, recalled that "she looked more like W. C. Fields" with her bulbous nose and doughy complexion.

Her manner was as severe as her appearance: stern, no-nonsense, intimidating to adults as well as children, and in charge. Burris recalled that the only time she saw her smile was during her first day in quarantine. "She and I jointly discovered that although I couldn't move any part of either my right or left leg, I could wiggle the big toe of my left foot." Her later contacts with the famous healer were all business, and the seven-year-old girl, as did all other patients, immediately learned to call her own "rear end" her "gluteus maximus."

By the mid-forties, though Sister Kenny had won many converts, the treatment of polio continued to be a matter of controversy,

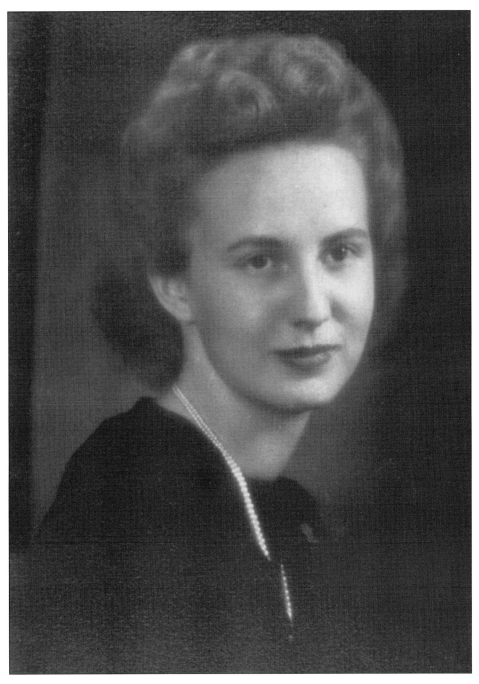

Virginia Royce, early 1946 (*Author collection*)

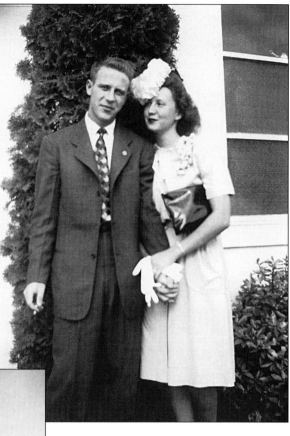

Del Black and Virginia Royce
on their wedding day,
September 13, 1946
(*Author collection*)

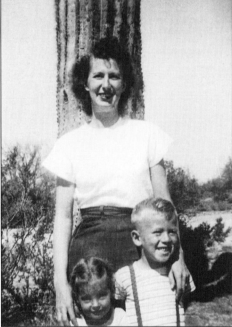

Virginia with Kenny and Kathy,
near Phoenix, c. 1954 (*Author collection*)

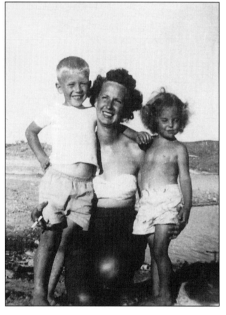

Virginia with Kenny and Kathy,
near Phoenix, c. 1954 (*Author collection*)

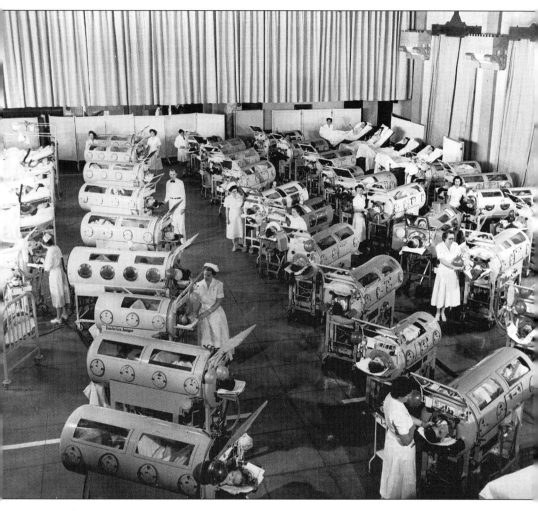

Rancho Los Amigos polio patients in iron lungs and on rocking beds, Hondo, California, December 26, 1952 (*March of Dimes Birth Defects Foundation*)

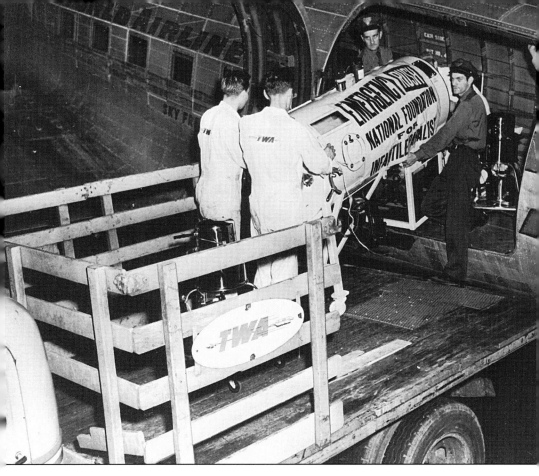

Iron lung being loaded into a
TWA plane at LaGuardia Field in New York,
bound for Kansas City, Missouri, 1950
(*March of Dimes Birth Defects Foundation*)

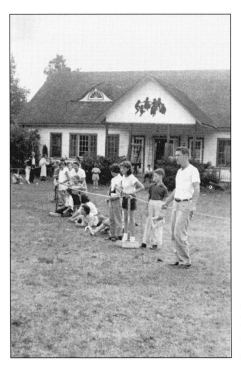

Campers and counselors in West Copake,
New York, separated from visitors to avoid
contagion, c. 1953 (*Manus Coen, photographer,
collection of Marion C. Katzive*)

since no one method had been proved more effective than others. Writing in *Harper's* magazine in 1945, Howard A. Howe, a neurologist and then the head of the Poliomyelitis Research Center at Johns Hopkins University, laid out for readers the three schools of thought. One group "hotly" maintained that rest was the important factor, saying weak muscles were sensitive to damage by overwork. That camp still advocated casting to hold joints in neutral positions. Followers of Kenny favored movement as soon as possible, which was hastened by hot packs. A third group insisted that patients with no treatment did as well as others. Howe came down in favor of movement, reasoning that even normal muscles tend to become fixed and less elastic if the joints aren't moved. Howe noted that so little controlled testing had been done that no one could say for sure what worked best; and such testing wasn't likely, because as soon as a new treatment became known, anxious parents insisted on its use.

In her efforts to publicize her cause and spread her ideas, Kenny often alienated others, especially physicians, with her sometimes arrogant and pompous style. Invited to lecture at a Washington, D.C. hospital, she arrived in a limousine, had a carpet rolled out for her, and had an escort into the auditorium. "She gave the impression she was a charlatan," William LaJoie, one of the Georgetown University of Medicine students in the audience, recalled. Nonetheless, LaJoie, like many others, came to consider her arrival in this country a "Godsend," and eventually became a physiatrist deeply involved in polio care.

Kenny, never a diplomat, accused orthopedists of being afraid that her methods would cut into their profits. She also resisted subjecting her methods to rigorous scientific testing, claiming that her word and recovered patients were enough. She further offended doctors by clinging to patently wrong ideas. Instead of sticking to what her clinical experience in Australia had taught her about treatment techniques, she went far afield and refused, for example, to believe that polio was a nervous-system disease. Also, she peppered her lectures with unscientific statements that made doctors cringe. She insisted that atrophy and paralysis came from failure to follow her instructions to the letter, rather than from actual cell damage.

Bitter struggles with the medical profession and the NFIP marred Kenny's last years. "Although the National Foundation had been ready and willing to take Sister Kenny under its wing . . . this was not the way that this powerful lady viewed the situation at all," wrote Paul. "Her hopes were that she might succeed in taking the NFIP under her own wing." A personal conflict between Kenny and the NFIP'S director Basil O'Connor—each, according to the Kenny biographer Victor Cohn, "unsatisfied, restless, a perfectionist, proud Irish"—stood in the way, but the conflict was primarily over power and control. Kenny called the short courses in the "Kenny method" sponsored by the NFIP, which lasted two to six months, "shoddy," insisting it took two years to learn her methods. She wanted control of the teaching, as did the NFIP, which argued that it had the funds, the administrative experience, and the support of the American people.

Kenny was called arbitrary, domineering and difficult—probably all accurate—and yet she was also self-sacrificing. She turned away financial rewards and even marriage to pursue, over her entire adult lifetime, the fight to get her methods accepted. No doubt she could have accomplished more by being more tractable, but then, wrote Cohn, "she would not have been Sister Kenny."

KENNY'S REGIMEN INVOLVED several time-consuming steps and required that nurses and doctors be retrained. She advocated that patients in the early stages of polio be put on hard beds with feet pressed against special foot boards to simulate standing, and physicians came to cajole children into the "polio position." She advocated hot, moist packs applied to painful muscles and daily warm baths, followed by an icy spray to stimulate circulation. Her muscle training, to be done daily, included both passive range-of-motion exercise (meaning a therapist moved those limbs and other muscles that were paralyzed) and an encouraging of patients to concentrate on the paralyzed part being moved, a technique similar to today's visualization.

The hot packs and physical therapy were soon common practice at hospitals and rehabilitation centers. Nurses and aides rolled in machines that looked a bit like ringer washers (and sometimes were) and plugged them in to heat up the water and blankets inside. Meanwhile, the patient was readied with rubber sheets on the bed. Nurses, physical therapists, or aides applied the packs, then sometimes covered them with more rubber sheeting and wrapped the patient with more blankets. The treatment, in the early stages, could be painful, but it could also bring a release from pain.

On the day he should have been starting school, fifteen-year-old Keith Dixon was being flown to a hospital in Regina, Saskatchewan, two hundred miles from the farm where he lived with his family. His hot-pack treatments began as soon as he arrived. He saw the nurse wince as she laid steaming towels on his body, and his whole body burned, inside and out. Each time, she asked, "Is it too hot?" And when he did flinch, she slowed in her work and waited until he could bear the heat again. She then left him, his body covered in the towels, and later she came back with her tub to lift them off, one by one. The air was fresh and cool against his damp skin, and that moment was the closest to relief he'd known in many days.

As the weeks passed, he learned to anticipate the hot compresses by the smell that preceded them—the hot, humid smell of wet fabric, which was more antiseptic than the hot laundry water at home. It was a paradoxical smell that meant both pain and relief were on the way.

Patients grew less tolerant of the wet and heat and disturbance, however, as the weeks and months of treatments went on. The joke among polio patients that "any pack too hot to hold was dropped on the patient" wore thin as, like Dixon, they came to dread the odor of wet wool and cotton flannel and the searing heat to come, sometimes with the whole process repeated every hour through a twelve-hour day. Sometimes nurses tied down the arms of children who insisted on ripping off the thick, itchy rags. In children's hospitals the cries of reluctant patients could be heard through the halls. Gertrud Svensson Stockton, a physical therapist, remembers that "the hot pack girls" always felt sorry for "the poor little patients" and had to be supervised to make sure the dressings were as hot as possible. Some children remember the experience as punishment: "The nurse would come in all the time and burn my neck with hot rags," was how one boy saw it. "At times it often seemed to be torture to us," said Jane Stevens, who was sixteen when she contracted polio in 1944, remembering her two months of hot packs that came as many as three times a day. "You were lucky if they were removed before they got too cold and started to itch. Imagine the smell of wet wool and sweat—this was summer in New Orleans," she remembered.

Patients endured the highly uncomfortable treatment; workers on the nursing staff endured the time-consuming, physically demanding task through years of polio treatment. Then doctors determined that hot packs were useful only in a few instances and only to relieve muscle spasm and pain, usually in the early stages of the disease. They did not, as hoped, prevent or cure paralysis.

In relieving pain, however, the hot packs did speed the patient toward the intensive, early physical therapy advocated by Kenny that proved so useful. Not only did her physical therapy strengthen weakened muscles and teach others to perform new jobs, but it also provided an important psychological boost to patients. Instead of lying immobilized, patients worked daily to regain function.

Whatever controversy there was over Kenny's method, most medical people agreed with the NFIP medical director, who listed these five points as the major benefits of her treatment plan: It relieved pain in the acute stage; it brought physical therapy promptly, thus minimizing contractures; it made the most of the muscles left intact; it provided constant and generous treatment; and it inspired hope and confidence in the patient.

After decades of trial and controversy, polio treatment settled into a regimen of rest and support for affected limbs during the acute stage, along with "freedom as far as possible from physical and mental trauma," according to Paul, followed as soon as possible by exercise and reeducation of muscles.

FOR MANY PATIENTS, CARE CAME in two distinct stages: acute care in a hospital and then rehabilitation, sometimes in a different location. For many, the shift brought dramatic changes. Leaving general hospital care meant leaving behind the deprivations of hospital life that came in many forms—prescribed food at prescribed hours, limited or no family visits, care from medical staff hidden behind the masks that reminded patients of their serious conditions. For many patients, acute care came in county or city general hospitals where patients with contagious diseases were sent. There, they might find cockroaches climbing the walls, or unappetizing food set on trays by their beds, but no one available to feed them. Doris Seligman found other particular discomforts at Willard Parker Hospital in New York. She was in a ward one floor below the tuberculosis patients, who spit out the screenless windows and left the polio patients below cringing at the thought of TB drifting into their open windows.

From the likes of that, many then entered a world where they no longer were considered sick, where the focus was not on merely keeping them alive but on getting them back into home life and the world. In rehabilitation they saw people dressed in street clothes instead of hospital white. They joined other patients in open wards where they could socialize and encourage one another. In acute care one could be lost in a sea of patients in desperate need, but in rehabilitation a team of caregivers—occupational therapists, orthopedists, physical therapists, social workers, doctors, nurses, and aides—all worked to bring improvements that would lead the patient home. In rehabilitation, patients, led by caregivers, had purpose, direction, and hope. For some, the feeling that they were making progress was all that kept them going through the painful and lengthy process.

The leading place in the country for polio rehabilitation and physical therapy was Roosevelt's Warm Springs, which came to be called the Little White House. Over time it sharpened its aim of giving aid to patients and to passing on to the medical profession useful observations or methods that might be used elsewhere. Medical workers from across the states traveled to Georgia for training in the care of polio patients. Gertrud Svensson Stockton, a physical therapist trained in New York City and working in Tennessee, traveled to Georgia for training there and once assisted FDR's regular physical therapist in one of the president's muscle evaluation sessions. She recalled that he contributed immensely to the morale of patients, doing his best to be one of them during his stays there. He ate with the patients and staff in the regular dining room and, although elsewhere Secret Service agents hoisted him to standing, at Warm Springs, like every other patient, he struggled with locking his leg braces and getting to a standing position on his own.

Staff, just like patients, had a sense of well-being and purpose at Warm Springs. Those in training attended classes in the morning, spent long lunch hours with patients and colleagues, rested after lunch, and then played bridge with patients and staff, as Stockton remembers it.

Patients, too, came from afar, some to have their residual paralysis evaluated for a treatment plan, some to get new braces or have surgery, some for extended physical therapy. Children and adults with a wide range of disabilities, though no respiratory patients, put in time at Warm Springs. Stockton remembers among the patients there during her postgraduate course were an engineer from Proctor and Gamble in Ohio, a Kentucky mother with a toddler and an infant at home, a soldier who had become sick in Africa, and the son of a French politician.

Warm Springs had an aura that drew respect—even reverence—from visitors, patients, and staff. Stockton remembers her stay there as "the absolute happiest time of my professional life." The special place Warm Springs held in the hearts of its devotees came in part from the poignancy that surrounded struggling, brave crippled children, but also from the importance it held in Roosevelt's life. Calling him "the world's most eminent statesman," a reporter for the *New York Times Sunday Magazine* gushed over the president and Warm Springs in an article called "Hope and Courage—That Is Warm Springs." The president attributed the spirit of Warm Springs to the Indians who years earlier had made the site a sanctuary for their wounded. That spirit, FDR said in a speech given there in 1934, "has been here at least as long as I have been here, and I am quite sure it will always rest on these buildings." The *Times* reporter went on to list in his article, which ran during the January 1944 March of Dimes drive, examples of the special quality found there.

> Take the case of a concert pianist whose hands were spared but whose feet were so affected that it was impossible for him to use the pedals of the piano. He has

turned painter and his watercolors are bright and beautiful. That is the spirit of Warm Springs.

Then there is the girl whom a doctor saw learning to walk.

"What is her muscle set-up?" he asked.

"Muscles? She hasn't any," he was told. "She walks with her head!"

And that is the spirit of Warm Springs.

Or the boy who could walk only on hands and feet. Determination put him through years of operations; then training here. Now he walks on crutches and holds a responsible position with a magazine in New York. That is the spirit of Warm Springs.

Ideally, rehabilitation began with doctors evaluating patients and making estimates about the potential recovery of muscle use and strength. They then prepared a treatment plan to be administered over months in the hospital and then, in many cases, for months following hospitalization. The physiotherapy process could go on for years, while patients learned to strengthen and make new uses of their available muscles.

Treatment followed one of three directions, depending on the condition of a particular muscle. With muscles showing complete or near-complete return of potential, bed rest, exercise, and overall good health formed the pattern. With a muscle showing partial return, strengthening of the less-damaged portions, training of undamaged muscles near the damaged one to compensate, and a long regimen of physiotherapy intended to bring some portion of a muscle's normal strength back were tried. With those muscles or muscle groups completely lost, physical training to prepare the patient to use supportive appliances, such as braces, was conducted.

Physiotherapists started by grading muscle strength using a "muscle chart" devised in part by FDR at Warm Springs, which gives a muscle-by-muscle evaluation of the body. Grades ranged from zero to five—meaning normal, good, fair, poor, and trace—with plus and minus grades given as well. At regular intervals during the sometimes lengthy therapy, patients listened anxiously to their marks, feeling sometimes discouraged, sometimes heartened by the incantation of "poor, poor-minus, trace, good, fair-minus," and so on.

Physical therapy and the physical therapist came to be the source and symbol of healing for patients. Teenager Jane Stevens had been hospitalized for three months, with her days consisting of little more than eating meals, having hot packs, reading, and getting ready for Sunday visits. Then the hospital hired a physical therapist, and "life was never the same," Stevens told me. "She had us exercising and learning to walk again. . . . Miss Lucy was our hero—she worked wonders with many of us."

The typical physiotherapy plan for a child with one leg paralyzed began with the therapists bending and manipulating the leg while the patient lay on a stretcher. The process might start with the child being able to endure no more than a half-inch lift of the leg from the table. That might be followed by hydrotherapy, in which the buoyant effect of the water might allow the child to move the affected leg more easily. Some patients could walk in the water, but nowhere else, and that in itself was heartening. Few hospitals had swimming pools, but as the epidemics wore on, many acquired pools of some sort. Some were large vats with slings to hold the patient suspended in the water while therapists manipulated their limbs. Some had deep tubs for walking; some even had wheelchairs that went into the water.

From water therapy the child with an affected leg might, over several months, progress from moving the leg to and fro while lying on a mat, to standing while being held, to walking up and down a ramp while he supported himself on armrails, to taking his first steps with the braces and crutches.

The *Saturday Evening Post* in 1949 ran a large photograph taken at Boston's Children's Hospital showing polio victims being taught "to carry out the activities of normal living in the functional training room." Three nurses in starched white oversaw the activities of four patients in an elaborately outfitted room. One, a grade-school boy with spindly arms and legs, rode, unaided, a stationary bicycle. A young girl, perhaps five years old, with braces on both legs and metal crutches, tried to step onto a subway car; a young man came down a flight of stairs; and a boy with bandaged, but not braced, legs walked with the aid of a nurse.

Patients did calisthenics, practiced with their wheelchairs and crutches, walked, swam, and received massages. And every small, day-to-day gain was cheered by the physiotherapist. In many, many cases the gains fell far short of complete recovery, but still the patients had a sense of progress. Dean Williamson, a young father of twenty-nine when he was severely paralyzed in 1955, gained strength slowly. He wrote of that time, "Just eating a meal was a problem; it took weeks of practice before I could feed myself without spilling. Each meal was an ordeal; my gown would become soaked with perspiration, and many meals were left unfinished for lack of strength to lift the fork. Therapy was beginning to show its benefits, though, for my neck and arm began to improve. As yet there was no indication of improvement elsewhere."

A BIG DAY FOR POLIO PATIENTS in rehabilitation came when they were fitted for braces. Mid-nineteenth-century orthopedists had known that supporting a paralyzed limb with braces or splints could not only help someone to walk but also prevent deformities. Being fitted for braces was regarded, according to Davis, not as a "sign of severe or permanent incapacity but as proof that they were getting well and were ready to go home."

Not everyone saw braces as a positive sign, however. One boy, an eleven year old who had been treated for four months before getting a brace, ascribed a curious, but apparently not unusual, meaning to the device. He reasoned that it was a sign of failure; as long as he was in bed, he thought he was improving. Once on the brace, he thought that was as far as he could go.

Braces came in all sizes and types. A two-year-old girl wore L-shaped shoes to keep her feet in the proper position while sleeping or resting. Mary Bready was first fitted with a "Toronto boot," a device like an open cast that supported her foot and bent knee. When the doctor came around to ask whether she was comfortable, her reply was, no, not entirely. It was too short for her long leg and the knee bent below her own. "A flurry of activity and I soon had the proper [fit]. That evening, the nurse in charge of the floor came by and said, 'Why didn't you tell *us* that you were uncomfortable?' And I said, honestly, 'I haven't been comfortable for so long that I didn't know I was supposed to be.' "

If a patient had extensive muscle damage, she might be fitted with a trunk brace, something like a steel-ribbed corset, that allowed her to sit up. Full leg braces brought the severely crippled to a standing position, but learning to use these devices required much practice. The writer Leonard Kriegel, who contracted polio when he was eleven, was fitted for double long-legged braces bound with a pelvic band circling his waist just before his twelfth birthday. "Lifeless or not," he later wrote, "my legs were precisely measured, the steel carefully molded. . . . It was technology that would hold me up—another offering on the altar of compensation." He described his first wearing of the braces that would become constant companions:

> After the steel bands around calves and thighs and pelvis had been covered over by the rich-smelling leather, after the braces had been precisely fitted to allow my fear-ridden imagination the surety of their holding presence, I was pulled to my feet. For the first time in ten months, I stood. Two middle-aged craftsmen, the hospital bracemakers who worked in a machine shop deep in the basement, held me in place as my therapist wedged two wooden crutches beneath my shoulders. . . . I stood on the braces, crutches beneath my shoulders slanting outward. . . . I flushed, swallowed hard, struggled to keep from crying, struggled not to be overwhelmed by my fear of falling.

Some of those newly fitted for braces saw the promise of new mobility and a return to home life, many shared Kriegel's fear, and almost everyone had to expend considerable effort to learn to use them. In addition to such major concerns, almost all but the youngest patients felt disappointed about the thick, sturdy shoes required by the braces. They represented one more barrier between the stricken and the hale, one more outward sign of difference. When white bucks and penny loafers were the standards for school, when young women longed for graceful shoes and girls for patent leather, the practical, clumsy footwear brought yet one more letdown.

Just before her polio attack, Mary Bready had gone shopping for a new pair of black dress pumps and had found a magnificent satin pair with three-inch heels and a pearl buckle. They had cost twenty-eight dollars—almost twice what she had to spend—and so she had settled for practical black leather pumps.

Later, in the hospital, looking down at her leg wrapped in a padded leather belt and braced between two steel bars that hooked into the leather heel of a heavy shoe, she remembered those satin pumps and wished with all her heart that she had bought them. She might have worn them only once, but at least she would have had that: one outing in the prettiest shoes she'd ever had on her feet. Now she was spending forty-five dollars for a pair of shoes that looked to her like a great-aunt's—black leather lace-ups with solid two-inch square heels. The heels had to be made of leather so holes for the braces could be drilled into them; normal heels wouldn't accept the brace, and low heels didn't offer enough room for it.

Orthopedic surgeons often stepped in along the way to correct or lessen deformities and handicaps left by the disease, by stiffening wobbly joints, reshaping bones, or transplanting usable muscles to more strategic locations, such as to a thumb or ankle. A common surgery for children with one withered leg was performed on the good leg to slow its growth. Otherwise, it could surge ahead of the damaged leg by several inches. Some patients had not one or two operations to correct a polio problem, but dozens over a decade or longer.

THROUGHOUT THE POLIO DECADES, but especially in the immediate postwar years, the orthopedists and the physiotherapists conflicted in their ideas about polio rehabilitation. The orthopedists advocated surgery, which had been an option since the later part of the nineteenth century when anesthesia and antisepsis came into use. The physiotherapists, newcomers who had gotten a tremendous boost from Sister Kenny, championed physical therapy.

The American Orthopaedic Association in the forties stood firmly against physiotherapy: "It is futile [and wasteful] to try to exercise muscles that are completely paralyzed or are so feeble that they have no functional value." Not surprisingly, they advocated surgery, saying: "The largest and most fruitful field of treatment of residual paralysis consists in the many orthopedic operations which have been devised to secure permanent correction of deformities and to improve the function of the extremities." Although many orthopedists privately doubted that physiotherapy did much beyond the natural recuperative processes, few pressed the point in actual treatment situations because they were aware, implicitly at least, of the valuable psychological functions it served.

For their part, physiotherapists did not rule out the possibility that paralysis could be so severe that physiotherapy would do little good, but they were optimistic about the potential benefits of a well-planned program of exercise and muscle reeducation. Physiotherapists contended that weakened muscles and those located near weak ones, over a long period of time, could be sufficiently strengthened to substitute or compensate for a functional motor loss. Many physiotherapists (and some patients) privately thought that surgeons performed far too many experimental operations in their effort to discover what worked and what did not.

One woman, grown protective of her quadriplegic husband through his months of hospitalization, watched with dismay as orthopedic surgeons operated on other severely handicapped patients. As she saw it, the most gullible, least-educated patients were operated on first in what she regarded as highly speculative, experimental surgeries. What seemed to be happening was that surgeons took a trace muscle, one with the slightest bit of movement, and moved it somewhere more strategic. In her observation, however, the procedure seldom worked.

One day she and her husband, a lawyer, were in conference with doctors at the hospital discussing the man's care when a surgeon explained that he wanted to do an operation that might allow the man to rotate his wrist. He declined the offer. The physician persisted. Again the patient said no. The surgeon went to the man in his wheelchair, picked up his limp arm, and dropped it alongside the wheel. "Look," he said, "can you get it back up?"

The patient, encircled by hospital staff, slowly, tediously crawled his fingers in a crablike way up the spokes of the wheel.

The surgeon watched, then said, "If I do this operation, and it works, you'll be able to eat soup with that hand."

"I'd rather sip from a straw the rest of my life," the man said, standing his ground against what he saw as surgical guesswork.

In my research, hunting for the breaking news on polio, I read issues of consumer science magazines of the forties and wondered whether the readers of fifty years ago felt as skeptical as I did scanning the frequent reports of new surgeries for polio patients. In 1941, for instance, a physician at the Crippled Children's Hospital in Marlin, Texas, determined that paralyzed muscles sometimes failed to work because of "bands of diseased tissue within the muscles." To repair the muscles, the doctor cut out the diseased bands or weaved through them strips of tendon from the bulky part of the muscles below or above the paralyzed one. He'd had success with six of twelve patients he'd operated on.

Another group of doctors obtained "encouraging results" with an operation called "neurotripsy," or "nerve-crushing operation." The theory there was that with old cases of paralysis, some three or four years old, the doctors could injure the nerve fibers and thus stimulate them to generate new nerve filaments. "As these grow into a weakened muscle fiber, these fibers . . . take on new life and vigor. If the branching is of large enough proportions, an increase in range of motion and muscle power can be demonstrated in the entire muscle group." The work was "experimental" but "encouraging enough to warrant further study and to make the method available to orthopedic surgeons throughout the country."

The conflict between the practices of orthopedists and doctors of physical medicine could sometimes be heated, but the researcher Fred Davis contended that despite the strong and conflicting opinions on which treatment was best, he and his colleagues in their "extensive review of the literature on polio rehabilitation" failed to come across conclusive evidence on the matter.

With or without these therapies, the road any patient took toward recovery was highly individual—dependent on what had been left to the person after the siege of the virus, on the willingness of the patient to work at rehabilitation, and on the skill of the doctors and therapists involved in his or her care. In treatment centers, the individual nature of the disease became clear. Children learned, after being on a ward for a while, that any group of patients was divided into "new polios" and "old polios." The "old" ones had had polio in the past and were back in the hospital for additional therapy or corrective surgery. Any new polio had to wonder whether he or she would be back as an old polio one day.

TREATMENT OF POLIO IN ALL ITS STAGES was costly, and millions of dollars to pay for it came from the NFIP. For all the worries a family singled out by polio might have, financial concerns seldom topped the list. By the late 1940s the NFIP had become the first national, private organization to pay hospital and medical bills for those who could not afford them, and the test was not poverty, but merely bills beyond a family's ability to pay. Brochures educating the public about polio prevention included the flat statement, "Don't worry about expense, if your doctor says it's polio." Instead, people were urged to contact a local chapter of the NFIP for help. Acknowledging that few families, even those with "substantial incomes," could meet the full cost, the NFIP assured the public that treatments would be paid "in whole or in part, if you can't pay them yourself."

Care for polio patients was costly. In the fall of 1949 the *Saturday Evening Post* reported: "The medical costs average $2,000 per case and sometimes run as high as $10,000. This is beyond the means of most families, and about 85 per cent of those stricken by polio have obtained assistance from the Foundation." That $10,000 at the high end turned into $20,000 or $25,000 as the epidemics wore on and patients, like my mother, moved into long-term care. The local chapter in King County, Washington, which includes Seattle, spent just over $100,000 for patient care in 1953. In 1954 the total was over $150,000. One boy, stricken when he was a toddler, racked up a $15,000 bill in two and a half years, and his care wasn't over yet. The annual costs for one polio patient who, like my mother, was paralyzed and on a respirator were close to $15,000. This was at a time when one could buy a house for under $10,000.

The polio years came long before widespread health insurance, which meant that few people who came down with polio were covered by insurance at all; and if they were, it was probably inadequate. Specific polio policies, typically five thousand dollars of coverage for a family for ten dollars a year, began to be popular in the mid-forties and could cover an uncomplicated polio case. But even that much coverage was far from common. One man who had polio as a boy and whose family had polio insurance remembers that a colleague of his father's said the boy's illness was "divine retribution" for the father having taken out a policy, instead, presumably, of trusting in God's care.

In 1954 the NFIP gave aid to 74,000 patients, 50,000 of whom were carryovers from the previous years' epidemics. At the end of 1954, a record 70,000 cases, including my mother, remained on the rolls. The NFIP paid for services and equipment across the whole range of needs: hospital costs, transportation to treatment centers, doctors' bills; equipment such as iron lungs, rocking beds, and hydrotherapy pools for hospitals; braces, wheelchairs, and other orthopedic appliances; and ongoing follow-up care. The NFIP also paid for household help when mothers came down with polio. While Mary Bready recovered in the hospital for three months, the NFIP chapter in Baltimore, where she lived, paid for a housekeeper to help her mother, who was caring for the Bready children. The object was to keep the family functioning as normally as possible, and for many families it worked. One mother of two toddlers in Seattle said that without such household help, she and her husband wouldn't have been able to keep their family together during her illness.

The procedure for a family struck by polio was to contact the local chapter, although the chapter often got to the family first, to arrange for assistance. The chapter then notified the hospital that payment, in full or in part, for the patient's care would come from the NFIP. The money was dispensed through local chapters, one for all but a few of the nation's four thousand counties.

That system of local distribution, which became a hallmark of the organization, took some years to come into being. Some chapters balked at the policy of sending half their collected funds to the national office, and at least one Michigan chapter held back spending money on its local cases of polio in order to make its funds last as long as possible. Donald Thurber, the NFIP's Michigan director, said: "It took quite a bit of convincing to get them to feel they were not alone, but were part of a giant pool the public had established for hard-pressed areas. . . . Eventually the . . . [c]hapter took the plunge and committed itself beyond its depth to care for a costly case or two. There was considerable skepticism that the Foundation would come through. When it did, the local people called me with expressions of joy and relief, feeling that they would not have to stand before a community they had betrayed."

The difference between what a complicated case of polio could cost and the amount a small county could raise could be staggering. An Arizona boy from the tiny town of Chinle in Apache County, a sparsely populated area in the northeastern corner of the state, contracted a severe case. By mid-1954 his nineteen-month treatment in Phoenix hospitals, most of it in an iron lung, had cost $22,000. His local chapter paid for part of his treatment, but the entire county annually raised only $3,000 in the January March of Dimes. In seven years Apache County couldn't collect enough money for that one child's care. The bulk of his bills were paid out of the NFIP's National Epidemic Aid Reserve Fund.

The NFIP not only paid directly for patient care but also coordinated and paid for the movement of both personnel and equipment to cities and towns faced with epidemics. In one week in 1949, for instance, the NFIP recruited seventy-one nurses and seven physical therapists and transported them, along with 171 respirators and 157 hot-pack machines, to epidemic trouble spots. When it became clear that not enough doctors, nurses, and therapists were knowledgeable in the latest techniques, the NFIP set up and paid for training them. The NFIP largely fueled the revolution to the Kenny treatment method, funding training courses in her techniques, but the breech between the two powers was firmly established before the forties were over.

THE NFIP, AN EXTRAORDINARILY SUCCESSFUL private philanthropy, received its money from the public, beginning with the first President's Birthday Ball in 1934, which brought in just over $1 million. In 1945 the organization collected nearly $19 million, and in 1954, $54 million. With the huge fund-raising efforts came a seasonal nature to the polio year. One could almost forget polio during the late winter and into spring, as the year slumbered through the months of few new polio cases. Then came June and the steep climb in the number of cases that climaxed in August or September. As fall came on, new polio cases declined, and polio receded from the public mind, until the second polio season—the fund-raising one—geared up. Come January of each polio year, the press, radio, and television once again ran heartrending and upbeat tales of polio victims (usually showing the success of polio rehabilitation), designed to open the wallets of the public. Newspapers, even such venerable ones as the *New York Times*, tugged at the purse strings of readers, exhorting them to give "generously" to the January March of Dimes. In January 1949, the *New York Times* pitched in by showing "then" and "now" photographs of former poster children. The 1947 poster child, Nancy Drury from Louisville, Kentucky, was a victim of the 1944 epidemic. With her 1949 photograph, the *Times* reported: "Today she is completely recovered, as is the case with more than 50 per cent of those stricken, thanks to progress in research, diagnosis and care, all heavily financed by the Foundation. Her illness 'is like a bad dream,' says her mother, Mrs. Frank Drury, 'now that her father and I watch her playing and walking as easily as any of her friends.' "

Around the country, newspapers urged their readers to give. An editorial in the 1950 *Seattle Times*, titled "More Cases Than Ever," announced the opening of the annual March of Dimes drive for funds.

According to the article, progress was being made in research to heal and prevent the disease, and, said the author, "these studies must be pressed forward at all costs." A newspaper columnist in St. Paul, Minnesota, climbed to the top of the City Hall Courthouse on January 5, 1954, and pitched a tent, "determined to stay until St. Paul and Ramsey County residents donate[d] a $10,000 'ransom,' " just part of the local $250,000 goal for the polio fund drive. Wearing "Arctic clothing" and brewing his coffee on an electric hot plate, he wrote his daily column from his rooftop camping site.

Such strong encouragement, coupled with the widespread public fear of the disease, effectively rounded up both dollars and volunteers. Merle Ross, the codirector of the NFIP's Colorado office in the 1950s, said that finding volunteers to lead the programs and events and run the county chapters was the easy part of his job. The "intense desire to get rid of polio" meant many people willingly stepped forward, and the issue of how much time was involved "never came up," Ross said. "What needed to be done was done." Even inmates in Colorado prisons got in on the drive when Ross took envelopes to them to be addressed for mail solicitations.

Volunteers, sometimes wearing blue lapel pins in the shape of crutches, raised money in numerous and often ingenious ways. Voicing what other NFIP workers knew also, Ross said that he learned that "people give in direct proportion to the frequency they are asked." The more the fund-raising activities, the more the money that poured in. Ten small "ask its," as he called them, brought in more than one giant event. Raising the money was "not hard," he recalled, mainly because the notion of appealing for small amounts was well conceived. No one demanded big sacrifices, just dimes. People were asked to give up a movie or a dinner out, a new hat or a week's worth of Cokes. And people showered the cause with their coins and dollars.

Schoolchildren had March of Dimes cards shaped as schoolhouses with slots for their dimes and test tubes just the right size to stack with more dimes. Their local newspapers encouraged them to save their "candy money to help some boy or girl walk again." No amount of money was considered too small to contribute. A Colorado bowling league collected $11.55 one night by demanding a contribution each time a member failed to make a strike or a spare. "Let everybody dance so that others may walk," said the chairman of a community dance with a one-dollar admission charge that went to the March of Dimes.

Throughout the country the January drives went on. A former polio victim walked across the state of Idaho to collect pledges. In Yakima, Washington, people paid a dollar for all the cakes they could eat in a flapjack-eating contest. Arizona teens by the thousands collected twenty-five thousand dollars by knocking on doors with three short, three long, and three short taps (Morse code for SOS) to signal their arrival. Arlington, Virginia, turned over all the dimes deposited in the town's parking meters during January to the polio foundation. In Washington State, members of the Bellevue Junior Chamber of Commerce operated a roadblock one evening during the 1955 drive. On the main street, the twenty-five members of the group asked cars stopped at a traffic signal to pay a fee to combat the toll of poliomyelitis. They collected $340, mostly in quarters (when a movie cost $1.25), and one giver handed over a five-dollar bill.

No plea for contributions was too maudlin. A dummy made of a diving suit, sitting in a wheelchair and wrapped with cloth was stuck with safety pins. Passers-by were asked to make a contribution and pull out a pin, to "Help get 'Polio Joe' out of pain." While such events proceeded through the month, other volunteers mailed out dime cards to their neighbors, and still others opened contribution cards, counted and rolled the coins in paper wrappers, and rushed the money to the bank.

Celebrities did their part for the NFIP. Hollywood stars, among them Barbara Stanwyck, Robert Young, Jane Wyatt, Bob Hope, and Cary Grant, took to radio and television to ask for money, as did politicians. To kick off the 1955 fund drive, Richard Nixon, then the vice-president, wiped windshields at a service station, after pulling up in a chauffeur-driven Cadillac.

Polio was such an easy draw that raising funds to combat it became a kind of public habit. One of the most successful national fund-raising efforts began as a local event for the Phoenix 1950 January March of Dimes. Calling it the Mothers' March on Polio, the

Phoenix chapter shaped the event, like so many other polio fund-raising efforts, around the basics of simplicity and communitywide involvement, touched with a dash of poignancy—in this case, supplied by the notion of mothers collecting to save children. The house-to-house solicitation, organized by elementary school districts so that volunteers worked their own neighborhoods, was given a novel touch by asking residents to leave a porch light burning as a signal to "marching mothers" that a contribution waited inside. No one would be solicited who didn't want to participate, but everyone, from the youngest and poorest to the well-to-do was asked to pitch in. The Phoenix organizer, in typical March of Dimes spirit, asked something from everyone, no matter how small the donation: "A gift of a penny from a family who can only place a candle in a bottle on their porch will be as welcome as a hundred dollars from a home with an elaborate porch light." Organizers made it easy on the volunteers, asking them to solicit for only one designated hour in the evening and asking that they carry only a "polio scroll" for contributors to sign.

In the week leading up to the porch-light parade, local newspapers encouraged readers to be home with their lights burning. Children were urged to dig into their pockets for a contribution and to sign the scroll themselves. One newspaper reminded readers: "The March of Dimes is YOUR campaign. It supports the program of the National Foundation for Infantile Paralysis, which protects YOUR child. If polio should ever strike your home, and we pray that it never does, the best of medical care is available IMMEDIATELY."

Volunteers rounded up almost $50,000 in that one hour of work, which was just $18,000 short of the previous year's total take for the entire county. Fifty volunteers, bank tellers and others, worked into the late hours of the night to count the collection. Chapter officials said the most amazing part was the number of follow-up calls from people saying no one had come to collect their money, even though they had waited, porch light shining, for a chance to give to the cause against polio. "We've never had so many folks begging us to take their money," said the county fund-raising director.

With success like that, other communities were eager to try the idea as well. In succeeding years, the Mothers' March became the climax event for the national January campaign and raised about 25 percent of each year's total take for the NFIP. In 1954, ten thousand Seattle women covered their city. Men, teens, and college students put on tags reading Tonight I Am a Mother and joined local mothers in the fund drive. One January, Merle Ross, with the Colorado office, dressed as a woman for the Mothers' March and enjoyed the good-natured ribbing he encountered from men on his route.

THE PROMISE TO PAY for the cost of patient care and rehabilitation dug deeper and deeper into the NFIP coffers. In 1949, reporting on the almost two hundred thousand dollars given to local chapters to cover treatment costs in one week, *Newsweek* warned of the threat such costs caused to the other important goal of the NFIP: research into the prevention and eradication of polio epidemics. If polio continues "in its present critical state," the magazine said, "it may be necessary to cut back on research funds to meet the immediate treatment needs."

By 1954, treatment costs ballooned to crisis proportions. Requests for emergency funds from chapters around the country were being met with payments of money borrowed from NFIP funds designated for research and education. And still the organization owed $2 million to the nation's hospitals. In the summer of 1954, Basil O'Connor pronounced the situation "serious" and designated the weeks of August 16 to August 31 as the time for an emergency fund drive to meet the critical financial situation. The record $54 million raised that January fell short of needs by $20 million. The country had heard often before from the NFIP that "never before in its history" was there a greater need for additional funds, and in 1954 they heard it again.

In June, the Maricopa County Polio Chapter in Arizona received emergency funds in the amount of $12,900 from the national office to help meet outstanding hospital, nursing, and other medical bills for the 152 patients in its care, including my mother. The chapter had already borrowed $17,700 from the national office in March after depleting local funds, and the needs kept mounting. By August the chapter was in debt more than $20,000 to hospitals, including $14,000 to Phoenix Memorial Hospital, where my mother lay in her iron lung.

In the midst of this financial crisis a volunteer from the Phoenix chapter approached my father, in what he remembers as an embarrassed manner, and "grilled" him as to whether he or his wife had any relatives with money to help in her care. He told them that none of his relatives had "anything" and as for her family, a few were "comfortable," but there was no reason they should be "broken financially" by her illness. Her summer of care had almost drained the five-thousand-dollar polio insurance policy, but Dad remained confident that the NFIP would take over when the money ran out.

On August 16, 1954, the emergency drive kicked off, and around the country communities gathered up the pennies, dimes, and dollars. This out-of-season drive, however, was met with objections from some local officials who worried that it would adversely affect other fund-raising efforts, especially "their local community chests," according to *Time* magazine. The news weekly reported that the Social Service Commission in Los Angeles first denied permission for the drive, and then "sheepishly reversed itself" when the local polio epidemic worsened. In Syracuse, New York, the local newspaper printed an angry editorial complaining that "far more money is raised for polio than cancer, heart disease or TB—which have higher death rates" and accused the NFIP of being "greedy and extravagant."

Most victims and their families received the considerable financial aid from the NFIP with gratitude. Betty Levin, who, with her husband, Alvin, had come down with the disease in 1955, called the organization "amazing, extraordinary." Payment, she said, was handled with the least bureaucratic interference; "they were forthcoming, kind, brisk, businesslike and efficient." One victim sent a letter to the editors of her local newspapers calling the NFIP "a life-saver to me and my family." "Without it," she wrote, "we surely would have been in debt for the rest of our life. Having this terrible disease is no fun at best, but I know beyond a doubt that my relief at learning my bills were being paid sped my recovery." But all that NFIP largess was not universally hailed. Some physicians, according to Fred Davis, questioned the "overindulgent policies toward polio families," seeing it as a precursor of socialized medicine and fearing that it "engendered lax and unappreciative attitudes in the families toward the medical care and treatment that the [patient] received."

And for all the financial help provided by the NFIP, many families, even those who were recipients of generous grants, still suffered financially. The organization could not and did not meet every need, and some needs fell outside its scope. What one occupational therapist called the "hidden costs of polio" included buying a new home or remodeling the old one to accommodate a handicapped family member, modifying or buying a new car, and hiring outside help for ongoing care. The Bready family, for instance, had stretched itself financially in July 1952 to buy an old, large house that could accommodate their three children and Mr. Bready's ailing mother. After closing on the $16,500 house, the young couple had $250 in the bank. "Being young and confident," said Mary Bready, "we figured we had nowhere to go but up." Her husband was an editorial writer for the *Baltimore Evening Sun*, and she had worked part-time in public relations. A month later, she was in the hospital with polio. The local NFIP chapter paid her medical bills, and the family took the aid gratefully. However, when Mary left the hospital with a brace on one leg, she was unable to drive their standard-shift car and had no money to buy an automatic. Before long, friends pitched in and helped the family buy a used station wagon.

My father tried, at first, to monitor the costs of Mother's treatment. He pored over hospital bills and questioned the insurance agent about items that seemed too high. He was particularly concerned about doctors who, in his view, had done little more than "stop by and say good morning" to Mother before putting through charges. Dad soon caught on to the system as he saw it, which was that money "poured" into the NFIP and into insurance agencies and plenty of people took advantage of that loose money. There was a lot of "stealing," Dad contended, "people being what they are." He quit worrying about money and trusted that someone else would pay the bills, which is what happened. He never felt he was taking charity, because he had contributed to the March of Dimes "like everyone else" and because he believed there was plenty to go around.

As costly as Mother's Arizona stay was, however, the bills would mount far higher as she moved from acute care to rehabilitation. Thousands upon thousands of dollars would go into special care, training, and equipment for her. Physical therapists educated in the methods of Sister Kenny and doctors specializing in the care of respiratory patients were standing by in Seattle, ready to help in whatever way they could. In those days, our family's prayers were for clumsy shoes and crutches, for a freely drawn breath, for miracles.

CHAPTER FIVE

Life Immobile

Sitting in the library one after-noon, scrolling through microfilms of the *Seattle Times*, I was reading the January 1955 issues. Because it was the March of Dimes month, I expected, and was finding, a good deal of polio news. When I saw a large photo of three women on the front page of the society section, I paused, my attention caught by a nurse's cap. I glanced at the caption and went cold as I read "Mrs. Delbert Black of Boulder, Colo., a patient in the hospital . . . "

As part of my search into my mother's polio years, I read old issues of newspapers, looking most carefully at those from Phoenix and Seattle. I wanted news of the disease in general, as readers forty and fifty years ago would have heard it and as major newspapers reported it, but I also wanted details from the specific places where my mother had been. My search of the Seattle newspapers was mostly for information about the Northwest Respirator Center. I wanted anything that might give me clues about Mother's life there. I had no memories of my own, as I had not been to Seattle with her, nor had my grandmother or brother. And when my father finished telling me all he could recall, there still were wide gaps in what I wanted to know. I didn't know what the hospital that housed the respirator center looked like, and no one there could find my mother's medical records, though her name is still in the computer.

I looked at the photo again. Mother was sitting reclined with her head resting against a chair back—a wheelchair, no doubt—her chest unnaturally small and lifted, a scarf concealing her neck and the tracheotomy hole I know was there. I studied her profile and saw my brother's nose. I had never known before that he had her nose. He looks so like my father in every other way it hadn't occurred to me that he had any of Mother's features.

In the photograph, Mother was smiling broadly into the eyes of the nurse, a pretty young woman who smiled back, her hand cupping my mother's cheek in a loving gesture. The third woman, who stood with a comb poised above Mother's head, was the chairman of the hospital volunteers. The caption said she had given Mother a permanent, with the assistance of the nurse, identified as "Miss Willa Dee Troester."

Alone in the dimly lit microfilm room, silent machines on either side of me, hunched forward with a notebook in my lap, I wept. I wept because I didn't recognize my mother, because the photo didn't show her to be as pretty as I'd thought she was, because I don't know my mother's face from memory. I recognize her only from photographs, none of which had ever shown me her profile. I wept in gratitude at seeing her genuinely happy smile and the tender ministrations of the two women near her. I wept, as I had so many times in my research, in surprise and disbelief at her helplessness. Again, forty years later, the knowledge that my mother had been devastatingly crippled came to me like fresh news.

On another day, I went back to the library, that time to search phone books and write down the addresses of every Troester I could find west of the Mississippi. I sent letters to them all, knowing the young nurse had probably married and changed her name, but hoping the letters that explained what I wanted would find a relative who knew where "Miss Willa Dee" was. I wanted to talk to her and find out whether she remembered my mother and whether she could tell me anything about Mother's experience at the Seattle hospital.

Later, at home, I studied the few photos of my mother I have, along with the grainy photocopy I'd made from the microfilm. I examined my own face in the mirror. My brother got her nose. Had I gotten anything? Once, recently, when I visited a high school classmate of Mother's to ask about her, the man said to me as I was leaving, "You favor her." "I do?" was all the response I managed. No one had ever said that to me before. My husband, Jens, and I pull out baby pictures of our mothers who never became grandmothers and lay them alongside those of our sons. And we see family. We see connections and the suggestion that something of our lost mothers has come back to us through our sons.

WEEKS PASSED AND I HEARD FROM NO TROESTERS, but in the meantime I found the names of the center's director, the physician Fred Plum, and assistant director, the physician Marcelle Dunning, and sent letters to them, too. Almost immediately I heard back from Dunning, saying she was willing to talk to me about her years at the Northwest Respirator Center. Not only that, she wrote, but she remembered my mother. She still knew Willa Dee Troester, too, and Shirley Wheeler Chiles, who had also been a nurse there, along with Elizabeth Wheelwright, the physical therapist, and Bertha Larsen Doremus, the social worker. In fact, a whole group of former patients, some of whom had been there at the same time as my mother, and staff were gathering for their annual potluck picnic next month. "Would you like to come?" she asked.

ON MONDAY, SEPTEMBER 27, 1954, Mother, in her iron lung inside the C-47, landed at the Boeing airfield outside Seattle and was met by an ambulance and representatives from the King County Chapter of the NFIP. Waiting at the hospital were Marcelle Dunning, Bertha Larsen Doremus, nurses, and attendants. The ambulance drove her through the city to Harborview Hospital, a ten-story blond-brick building from the thirties that sat on a hill overlooking the Seattle seaport. I suppose Mother, in her iron lung, entered by way of the ambulance door, rather than through the street-side public entrance, elegant and ornate with its marble and brass. I wonder whether in 1954 she noticed, as I did on the day I visited there with Dunning in 1994, the sounds from below—foghorns, boats calling to one another, cars on the highway. Harborview, a public facility used as the teaching hospital for the University of Washington Medical School, had never been as luxurious as some private hospitals, but it had excellent facilities, a grand appearance, and a dramatic location. Today, like many other public hospitals that once took polio patients, it houses many AIDS patients.

Seeing that stately building on a hill and knowing the respirator center was on the back with the water view heartened me. I know I would have found solace in both the beauty and activity that could be taken in from those windows, and I hope Mother did. Patients could watch trains load and unload cargo from the ships docked at the waterfront. A Standard Oil tanker from Alaska, an American troopship returning from Japan, unidentifiable freight sailing ships, and graceful passenger sailboats would have composed her view in those days. To the north was the Seattle skyline, then dominated by the forty-two-story Smith Tower, and in the distance, across the bay, Whidby and Bainbridge Islands and the snowy mountains of the Olympic Peninsula. From those windows, too, spectacular sunsets spilled into the hospital rooms.

On the day Mother and her tank were carried in, the staff saw with relief that her trip had gone smoothly. The flights didn't always. One woman had arrived so seriously short of oxygen that she was blue, either because the respirator had failed or because no one on board had known how to operate it. Seven patients watched Mother's arrival. Three were newcomers also, having arrived from Alaska together on a special flight three weeks earlier. They were a five-year-old boy, a thirty-two-year-old woman, and Molly Snyder, thirty, a Native American from the Aleutian Islands who had never before left her Alaska home. Her husband, a longshoreman, came with her, while their fifteen-year-old daughter looked after the five younger children at home.

When Mother arrived, the center—which was nothing more than a laboratory, an office, and two large, gray-walled hospital rooms, numbers 405 and 409—was already crowded. The seven patients and the complicated and bulky apparatuses that kept them alive filled the two patient rooms. There were rocking beds high off the floor with giant labels identifying them as belonging to the March of Dimes, rolling tables jumbled with medicines and gear, food trays, empty iron lungs waiting for patients who needed them at night, and all types of wheelchairs. To the side stood apparatuses to measure breathing, complete with gauges and dials and graph paper, tanks, hoses, and mouthpieces. In the next year, the hospital turned over one more room for patients and two others for physical and occupational therapy.

ON THE DAY OF THE GATHERING of the "Polio Alums" in Seattle, Marcelle Dunning drove me to the home of Janet Steputis, whose husband, Hank, had been the unit's first patient. There at the well-kept, one-level home with lush gardens and a large backyard shaded with two huge trees, I met people who had cared for my mother, suffered with her, remembered her. I felt like a distant cousin stepping into an ongoing family reunion. One of the first people I saw was Willa Dee Troester, whom I recognized immediately: her finely shaped features, warm eyes, and bright smile were hardly changed by the years.

Another nurse, Shirley Wheeler Chiles, handed me a package of papers, photos, and news clippings when we met. She flipped through them, in particular pointing out issues of "The Vital Capacitor," a mimeographed newsletter created and written by the center's patients themselves. Shirley had thought to mark each page that mentioned my mother. I couldn't believe my eyes. Here was a glimpse into the life Mother had led as a paralyzed patient. Answers to questions I had about what patients did each day, who was with her, what the place looked like, and more were there, not filtered by memory but recorded at the moment. Unable to wait, I stood in the sunlight and began to read immediately. Along with the particulars of their daily lives and activities, the patient-writers provided regular reports on the weather. For August: "Old Sol is on vacation!" For November: "Well, what did you expect . . . sunshine?" For February: "Still Raining." Those nutshell reports made me smile, just as I'm sure their original readers did.

And what I wanted most was there, too: news of Mother and articles dictated by her. In one, published in the fall of 1954, she told of arriving in Seattle:

I was impressed with . . . the friendly, easy atmosphere given by both patients and nurses. The Center differs from the hospital I was in in that . . . [e]verything is centered around each patient's needs. Doctors, nurses, physiotherapist, and the occupational therapist, as well as the many others . . . here are working together not only to re-educate or strengthen muscles, but also to provide recreation and education so that one's mind is occupied [and] he doesn't have to lie with nothing to do.

Mother's first couple of days there were given to evaluations. With each newcomer, the staff tested muscles and determined what the patient could do physically. Because all the patients needed help with breathing or swallowing or both, an important part of the evaluation was the patient's respiration. The doctors measured vital capacity, which is the size of the biggest breath out following a breath in, as one might do when given a single chance to blow up a balloon. They checked whether the person could take even a breath or two unaided and determined what muscles the patient used for breathing.

The social worker, Bertha Larsen Doremus, did a psychosocial assessment, looking for the effect of the patient's disability on both the patient and the family. She called herself "the connecting link" between the patient, the family, and the medical staff. Ordinarily, she interviewed the family members who accompanied patients, as well, but Mother arrived alone, out of context, with no one to add to what she could say about herself and her family.

The physical and occupational therapists did evaluations, too, looking for existing or potential skills, and then the entire staff convened to discuss the patient's future. From that first day, the ultimate hope for everyone was discharge to a home and family ready to provide care. The staff set intermediate steps toward that end and then monitored each patient's progress in weekly staff meetings.

Based on the patients' vital capacity, along with, as Dunning said, "what you had a hunch they could do," the staff set goals. For Mother, the aim was the most basic. It was, as Dunning told me, "to get her out of that tank." The day she arrived in Seattle was her 100th in an iron lung, and she had, in that time, become dependent on it physically and emotionally. Getting her breathing in some other way would be a major step in her rehabilitation.

At the Northwest Respirator Center, the policy was to wean patients as quickly as possible, at least for daytime hours, because the longer patients spent in a tank, the harder it was to get them out. Even while a patient was in the acute stage of the disease, which was spent in another ward of the hospital, staff from the respirator center consulted with doctors about what could be done safely to help the patient breathe without the confining machine. Then as soon as the acute phase had passed, ten or twenty days usually, the patient went right into the specialized unit for rehabilitation. When the center opened, Fred Plum was quoted in the *Seattle Times* saying: "If we have to wait until the patient has been in a hospital six or eight months we are behind the eight ball. . . . [Often] we have to convince the patient that he really is capable of facing life again. It's pretty hard to make someone who has been in a hospital six months realize he isn't really sick."

Mother arrived in Seattle behind the eight ball. Although she hadn't spent six months in the iron lung, she had been in it long enough to make weaning her very difficult. Most iron-lung patients, usually early in their care, improved enough to begin breathing on their own or with other mechanical devices, though the course each took was highly individual. A few people, however, couldn't do it, blocked by physical or emotional barriers, or both. Mother had little reserve in her lungs, little voluntary muscle control of any type, and whatever breathing muscles she did have had lost elasticity and strength in the months since the onset of paralysis. The staff had seen other tough cases, though, and had helped them. They would see how far Mother could go.

THE WEANING BEGAN with decreasing the pressure in the tank to see whether Mother's lungs could take over inside. Eventually the respirator was turned off, maybe only momentarily, to further test her. All along, the doctors assured her that she would not be forced beyond her abilities, and still they kept encouraging her to take voluntary breaths, even one or two.

The aim was to teach Mother to breathe on the rocking bed. Developed in 1947, this is a hospital bed that pivots by electrical power from head to toe, forcing air in and out by gravity. When the person's feet go down, gravity pulls the internal organs down, bringing air into the lungs; and when the feet go up, gravity pushes the organs against the diaphragm, forcing air out. The speed and depth of rocking are adjusted to the individual's needs.

Getting onto a rocking bed offers advantages both to patients and to those caring for them. The movement of the beds, which are still used, not only allows the paralyzed person to breathe, but provides a kind of exercise, reducing stiffness and muscle contracture. As the bed tips up and down, the body shifts as it cannot in the iron lung. The rocking also helps with blood circulation and bowel movement and with preventing calcium deposits and stones.

The move to a rocking bed, a joint effort of patient and doctors, took time and energy. "Those were scary times," Dunning recalled. Mother's progress was slow, hindered not only by her severe physical limitations but also by her fear. Surely she must have hated the tank for the claustrophobic existence it imposed, yet it kept her alive. As long as she was in the tank, she was safe; without it, who knew what might happen to her? She may have been held back, too, by memories of near suffocation. Nearly anyone who had been in an iron lung could tell tales of being stranded without breathing help. One such story was told by Gene Roehling, a teacher who had spent two years in an iron lung in California hospitals and who related his experiences in the *Saturday Evening Post* in 1951. Roehling told of having twice passed out from no oxygen, both times because nurses left open the big door to his respirator too long, in what he called "those lapses of mental process which will be forever unexplainable." The first time occurred when a nurse opened the door and simply left the room. The second time, a different nurse was giving him an enema and just stood beside him with the door wide open. "While she stood within twelve inches of me," he wrote, "I had those few uncomfortable seconds when I was short of breath, and then I was gone." Something broke the woman's reverie, and she slammed the door shut and saved him. Little wonder patients held captive by their immobility were fearful.

I wish I knew what Mother's first moment on a rocking bed was like. I suppose it was at once exhilarating and terrifying. After days, weeks, or months of being flat and immobile in an iron lung, patients often became dizzy from the motion. Mother's first time out might have lasted only a few minutes before she was returned to the womb of the tank, but the weaning went on with the persistent caregivers encouraging and reassuring, with other patients in view rocking, breathing, and living without the tanks they had once depended on.

To make sure the rocking gave the patient enough oxygen and eliminated enough carbon dioxide, Dunning analyzed blood from an artery. Using a syringe, lined with an anticoagulant, she penetrated a thick artery wall, usually in an arm, and drew blood without taking in outside air. The time-consuming, costly, and somewhat painful procedure might have been performed daily while the patient learned to use a new breathing machine. Writing for "The Vital Capacitor," Mother remarked on "the wonderful service" provided for all who needed the respirator center's care. "I must say, though," she added, "that no one has been so thoroughly examined or 'stuck' in only one week as the new arrival in the Center."

Gradually, Mother spent hours at a time on the rocking bed, which for her moved in a deep, full swing almost to the floor, a sign to anyone watching that she needed maximum aid with breathing. Others with more power of their own rocked more shallowly. No longer enclosed in the tank, she must have experienced a boost in morale. Now, instead of seeing only what was reflected in the mirror above her head, for the first time since coming down with polio, she could see across an entire room or out the window or down the hall from the gently swinging bed. Still dependent on an electrical cord for breath, still confined to a single room, still unable to move so much as a finger, she did at least have the freedom to shift her eyes and lay them on a variety of scenes as they passed before her. I wonder whether she tried to look down at her own body—or up at it as her feet swung above her head—and whether she was surprised at its thinness and awkwardness, her limbs placed in position rather than moving naturally.

The rocking bed offered additional comforts, such as a real mattress instead of the hard, narrow cot of the iron lung, and the bed's motion could have a lulling effect and induce sleep. I hope Mother slept, really slept, on her rocking bed. Out of the iron lung, whatever muscles might still be alive were encouraged to move, and staff could more easily tend her body with baths and physical therapy treatments. She could now be dressed each day and speak to others more easily, without the competing noise of the iron lung. She did, however, still have to measure her conversation in short phrases timed with the out breath and the swing of the bed. And her voice had no power; no loud shouts, powerful sneezes, or laughter came from patients with paralyzed breathing muscles. "When I laugh I do so without making a sound," wrote Arnold Beisser. "I have the internal experience . . . ; my face and body motions reflect that I am laughing, but no sound is emitted."

The weaning continued, with periods on the rocking bed and reprieves in the iron lung to relax. But the doctors pressed on to the next step for Mother, which was to adapt to the portable chest respirator, a kind of minilung that fit tightly over the trunk of the body and sealed to it. A black rubber hose connected it to a pump. The respirator worked by alternately pressing on the chest and lifting to bring air in and out. One woman said of her first experience with one: "The pressure made it feel as though my stomach were being pressed down against my backbone each time the machine 'inhaled.' I stood exactly 43 minutes of this, part of which time I bitterly wept—then returned to my lung with relief!" She tried again the next day at a lower pump pressure and lasted two hours and fifteen minutes. A while later the doctors decided she could try sleeping with it; she slept little and woke exhausted and eagerly returned to the "old tin can."

The chest respirator punched on the chest and squeezed against the flesh around the rib cage about eighteen times each minute, creating friction. Although, with proper padding, most patients adapted, they came to trade discomforts, alternating between the chest respirator and the rocking bed. When the fanning of air on tender skin began to irritate and the shifting weight of leaden limbs created painful pressure points, the patient went back to the chest respirator. Over several weeks, the staff worked with Mother until she could spend her nights on the rocking bed and her days alternating between the bed and being in a wheelchair with the Monaghan portable respirator breathing for her.

Writing for "The Vital Capacitor" a report that sounded overly calm to me, but in keeping with the positive tone of each issue, Mother said the rocking bed "was new and interesting," even if hers did stop a time or two during the night and "cause a little excitement." In the same issue one of the departing patients wrote a mock will, leaving to Virginia Black "a trustworthy Monaghan." Reading between the lines, I can readily see that her weeks of weaning were punctuated with episodes of near suffocation. I imagine her fear through feeling my own for her. And, yet, she pressed on and in two months was free of the iron tank.

WHEN DAD ARRIVED IN NOVEMBER, he saw Mother out of the iron lung for the first time since that June morning he had taken her to the doctor in Phoenix. A cataclysmic event had shaken their marriage, an eruption that would have shaken even the sturdiest of marriages, and theirs wasn't one of those. Digging into my parents' early years, the before-polio years, has told me much I didn't want to know about the unhappiness they brought to one another. I think it was a passionate marriage with emotions running high, and I want to think the bad times were balanced by good, but I'm not confident they were. From the beginning, their hasty marriage in Portland was rocky. Dad attributed it to "too much poverty and too different personalities." Early in the marriage, Mother left Dad a time or two and returned to her parents' home with Kenny, and when I was born, at the end of 1949, we all lived there. What had become of the home my parents had had, I don't know. What they felt for each other then,

I don't know either, but from what my father has told me, in the next four years, before polio found us, nothing happened to mend the wounds of those first few years. All I know is that the marriage was blighted, but they were still together.

Even if Dad had been eager to see Mother, his arrival in Washington couldn't have brought him much happiness. He had left Arizona reluctantly, something he attributed to the drastic change in weather, a switch as he saw it "from the best climate in the world to the worst." He loved the dry, sunny heat of Arizona and the constant opportunity it provided for being outside. He drove into Seattle in our Chevy on a day of fall rain that settled on him like depression. "I thought I had driven into the tail-end of the world," is how he remembers it. He found a job quickly, working as a collections manager for a loan company at $340 a month. He told his boss why he was in Seattle, but after that no one at the office discussed my mother. Dad did his job and at the end of the day stopped at a café for a sandwich before going to the hospital to see Mother. He couldn't cook for himself, as he lived in a single room without a kitchen, a couple of blocks from the hospital. But from the day of his arrival it was the weather, he said, that really brought him down.

The complicated history my parents shared must have colored their reunion in Seattle. But now that Mother was out of the iron lung, Dad could, at least, hold her hand. Perhaps he was pleased with her progress, but I know, because he has told me so often, that he never believed she would recover.

Perhaps he left Mother at the rehab center each night and returned to his single room to pray, as he had in Phoenix, for the death of one of them. That's a prospect that haunted me as I met more and more families touched by polio. In Seattle that summer so many years later I visited the polio alums, I talked to a man whose father had been as severely affected as Mother. He said that his mother, in those desperate early weeks when no one knew whether his father could survive, had "insisted" that he live, and he had. Playwright and author Charles Mee, writing about his encounter with polio, told of his father calling in a priest while Charles lay critically ill in the hospital. "Why did my father not tear down the walls of the hospital, scream at all the priests to stay away, shout to the world that his son would live, damn it, or he would curse God and all creation forever?" he wrote. "Why had he not staked everything on life for his son, gambled all for that life? Why not?"

I understand that man's thinking, because the same rage rips me. My father begged for a way out instead of insisting, willing Mother to live. I believe my father when he says, in Seattle, he was trying to do well by Mother, not just going through the motions expected of him by convention. I believe him, and still I wish he had behaved differently.

THE NORTHWEST RESPIRATOR CENTER, like the country's seven others that had come before it, was founded for the express purpose of rehabilitating polio patients, like Mother, with respiratory difficulties. Before the specialized units came into being, respirator cases were scattered in general hospitals throughout the country, sometimes just one or two to a hospital. In a health-care system that intends to cure patients and send them on their way, the kinds of chronic and severe problems that face people severely handicapped from polio, or any other source, are seen as a failure. The respirator centers became a place for patients to go and be seen, as Dunning said, not as sick people but as disabled people in need of rehabilitation.

The first aim of the specialized units was to free patients as much as possible from respirator aids so they could go home, which not only improved their lives but cost far less than hospital care. Center workers also conducted research in respiratory treatment, operated their facilities as laboratories for the evaluation and development of respirator equipment, developed teaching and consulting services in the care of the patients, and traveled to national meetings to share with other centers what they had learned. Baltimore was home to the first one, opening as an experiment in 1946 and showing clearly that group care meant better care for respirator patients. The NFIP soon funded four others, in Wellesley Hills, Massachusetts; Houston, Texas; Ann Arbor, Michigan; and Buffalo, New York. By 1952, three more, including the one in Seattle, were in the planning stages.

Grouped together, respirator patients encouraged and stimulated one another. A writer for the *Saturday Evening Post* in 1952 told of the first two patients to arrive at the Mary MacArthur Respirator Unit in Boston when it opened in 1950. They were two teenage girls who had spent months in the same hospital but had never seen each other. When they were wheeled into the new ward, nurses put the heads of their iron lungs together, adjusted the mirrors and introduced the girls. They took a look at each other's reflection and burst into tears. Said one, "I think we were crying for joy . . . because we'd each found a friend."

By national standards, the Northwest Respirator Center, set up to take a maximum of twelve patients, was small; others could handle several dozen. Now that I've met some of the people who were there with my mother, I'm grateful she went to Seattle for rehabilitation. I've seen for myself the camaraderie and good cheer of the former patients, the dedication of Marcelle Dunning and the affection and respect her former patients hold for her. I've looked into the gracious and affable eyes of Miss Willa Dee Troester, and I've been comforted by it all.

Staffed by the University of Washington School of Medicine and the Harborview Hospital, the Northwest Respirator Center operated with grants from the NFIP. It opened as the country's eighth center on November 19, 1953, intending to serve patients from the Northwest, Alaska, and Hawaii, although it eventually took patients from other states as well.

Fred Plum, now the chief neurologist at the New York Hospital Cornell Medical Center, was recruited in 1953 while still in the navy by the University of Washington Medical School. A scientist with a philosophical bent and an interest in people, he was unquestionably the commander-in-chief, keeping his focus on the patients under his care and on the research going on there that could benefit patients around the country.

Early in the setup of the Northwest Respirator Center he hired Dunning to work as his part-time associate director. The two then hired a staff, set up research programs, and traveled to other centers to meet with other directors and study procedures and explore problems.

While Plum had his eye on the big picture, Dunning, who was intimate with each patient's daily lab reports and was on the floor for rounds usually twice each day, kept the day-to-day operations going. She also kept close to the progress of the research projects. Like Plum, she was unflappable and smart, but both her role and her manner were different from his. Ambitious, focused, and in command, Plum was highly respected by his staff and patients. Such seriousness, intensity, and power in a young man set him apart and left an impression on others. He wasn't at the reunion picnic I attended in Seattle, and, in fact, had long ago lost contact with his former colleagues and patients. But he showed up vividly in the memories and stories others told. Patients spoke of him in such terms as "everyone was afraid of him," and "he was next to God," as they told stories of their willingness to approach him, despite his forbidding manner, and of his willingness to listen to even the lowest-level staffers.

Diminutive and quick, Dunning was professional but approachable. In my visit with her, I found her not given to motherly sentiment, but still deeply caring, as evidenced by her efforts even in retirement to keep up with former patients. When she was hired, she was near the end of a ten-year treatment of tuberculosis. Her personal experience with invalidism and long confinement in a sanatorium gave her an empathy for her patients not common among physicians. Word of her illness spread through the patients and helped bind them to her, one woman told me, though it was not something widely discussed.

As part of its mission, the Northwest Respirator Center trained residents and interns from the University of Washington. Each intern rotated to the unit for a month, and each resident, for three months. And each medical student spent three days there. Dunning made sure that each one climbed into an iron lung; she'd then turn the pressure so high he couldn't breathe with his own muscles. "I wanted those young and healthy people to understand the fear and panic that went with being in the tank," she told me. The students, she recalled, often were afraid to get in the iron lung and joked about it and teased each other. As a prank, a group once followed through on the often-voiced threat to leave someone inside, and Dunning came upon an alarmed young medical student who had been confined about fifteen minutes.

The center had opened with Plum and Dunning, along with residents in medicine from the University of Washington, Troester as the charge nurse who hired and trained a nursing staff, two lab technicians and others at the university's department of neurology to help with research, an occupational therapist, a physical therapist, a social worker, and a public schoolteacher provided by the school system. There was also a team of consultants: orthopedist, psychiatrist, obstetrician-gynecologist, and pediatricians available as needed. Dozens of professionals and a corps of volunteers, with all the equipment they needed, stood by to treat twelve patients.

WHEN MOTHER ENTERED the Northwest Respirator Center, she joined a community of young adults, teens, and children bound in common purpose and experiences. It was an active setting where children had their school lessons, students studying medicine and physical and occupational therapy came in and out, and family members visited daily. Volunteers came in to write letters for patients, take them for wheelchair walks, shop for them, and read to them.

The group was close-knit—like "a big family" was the phrase I kept hearing at the August picnic. The staff worked as a team, with even student nurses and orderlies involved in the conferences about patients. The organization was common to these specialized units, though not to regular hospitals. Plum's attitude was that, he said, "there wasn't much point in talking about patients without having the people taking care of them involved. I knew who was saving those people's lives and getting them home and it wasn't me."

The aim was for each staff member to have a well-rounded understanding of what each patient needed, medically, psychologically, and socially. Each person involved in the patient's care and rehabilitation reported impressions and information about the individual's progress. They worked together to help each patient with whatever essential skills he or she needed—swallowing, drinking, eating, breathing—and from there, whatever else the person might learn to do. It was hard duty. A study done at the Mary MacArthur Respirator Unit showed that even personnel who had enthusiastically volunteered for such work were sometimes discouraged by the strong emotional demands made by their patients' care. An attitude of "firm encouragement," the researchers found, was the most beneficial to the patients, as was acceptance of the patients in spite of their considerable emotional and physical limitations.

For each patient, living around the clock in one or two rooms with other people not of his or her choosing surely made for some difficult times, but the proximity and common problems also drew the patients into an unusual intimacy. Side by side, respirator patients provided comfort, encouragement, and community for one another. Norma Duchin, writing about her hospitalization elsewhere with other iron-lung patients, said: "The feeling of not wanting to be less brave than the person in the next bed was followed by the feeling of honestly wanting to be considerate and helpful. Then, slowly, mercifully, humor and affection grew. We became friends." The patients at the Northwest Respirator Center, like those Duchin lived with in Baltimore, continued over the decades to keep in touch, a testament to the gains they had made in each others' presence and to the deep bonds of friendship they had formed. It was obvious to me that the experience of being together through what was for most of them, no doubt, the greatest struggle of their lives had bound the Seattle patients as it had Duchin and her ward mates.

When teenager Shirley Winge was discharged from the Northwest Respirator Center in the fall of 1954, her "Last Will and Testament," appeared in "The Vital Capacitor." She began, "I Shirley Winge, alias Shirl, being of as sound a mind as possible considering my surroundings . . . " and then went on to bequeath something humorous to each staff member and patient. Dunning, for example, was given "one empty syringe and no small veins," and Troester was bequeathed "one old sterling silver trach tube." In that issue and every other, humor and goodwill were evident, and I'm cheered to know my mother was part of it.

Patients joked among themselves and with the staff, often with the dark humor common in difficult situations. Quips about the power going off and about bedpans and urine jugs, enemas, and visits with the consulting psychiatrist bounced around the rooms. As an orderly who came on duty in the evenings remembered it, "The cajoling and conversation kept going all the while like a Ping-Pong game until the patients went to sleep." And always, along with the banter was affection. Writing in "The Vital Capacitor" about the three-year-old girl who shared his room and was leaving, one man said:

> Jody and I carry on lengthy conversations as to the nature of our current meal and our progress in consuming it. It isn't the usual type of dinnertime conversation, but the friendly competition which causes us both to eat more. (For us, that's to be desired.) Yes, I'll miss that small voice piping up with 'Dick, have you finished your juice?' . . . Yes, after Jody leaves, every time I whistle for some much needed bagatelle, I'll miss her reassuring, 'Nurse be here soon, Dick,' or if the need was hers, Jody's earnest request to 'Whistle, Dick!' "

Looking back at the group of patients who received care at the center—106 in its short life from 1953 to 1958—Dunning noted that though the patients were young people of varying ages and interests, all but four or five were avid outdoors people, who liked being active and had little time or energy for contemplative activities before getting polio. "Physical activity was for them a way of dealing with stress," she said. There's no telling what giving up those activities entailed for individuals, but in the respirator unit they did, at least, have a social life. Patients and staff celebrated, as a big family would, births, birthdays, weddings, and holidays as the months and years passed. And each departure meant a party, as well.

Hungry for details that might put me there and let me imagine a celebration, I read in the newsletter the listings of those parties, but I found nothing more than a mention of the group playing a word game or being entertained by performers from a local variety show who had come to tap-dance and twirl batons. I learned that the group listened to lectures by instructors from the Cornish School of Allied

Arts on drama, art, and color, and that a women's sorority showed monthly sixteen-millimeter movies. Mother wrote under the headline "Society" and enumerated the social activities and the birthday and farewell parties, but "We all had such a nice time" was as deep as the commentary went. Aching to know what she truly thought and felt during those months in the Seattle hospital, I found her reports frustrating. At first, it seemed I had so much of her in front of me— actual words written by her at the time of her illness—but then nothing she wrote told me anything about what her days meant to her. Her language, mannered and distant, doesn't bring her into focus. Her stories weren't funny or irreverent or lively, as those of some others were. The lightheartedness so evident in the three letters I have that she had written from Phoenix was gone.

NOVEMBER 1954, TWO MONTHS after Mother's arrival, brought the excitement of a baby born to one of the patients. Marylin Angell had been pregnant with her second child when she got polio in New Mexico and was transferred to the Northwest Respirator Center in July 1954. Her husband and two-year-old son moved to Seattle with her. She progressed rapidly, moving to the rocking bed from an iron lung and gradually increasing her vital capacity and ability to breathe unassisted. Two weeks before her scheduled cesarean section, she aspirated fluid while on the rocking bed and would have choked to death had a surgical resident not been passing by at the time. She recovered sufficiently for the scheduled birth and delivered a healthy six-pound, one-ounce boy, whom the couple named James Emerson Angell. He's the child bearing the name *Emerson* in honor of the tank that had saved Marylin's life. What all this—Marylin's near-death right before their eyes, then the miracle of a healthy baby born in the midst of her severe illness—did to the other patients, my mother among them, I can't know. Their days were measured in routine and tedium, and yet there in the person of Marylin was a reminder of both the nearness of death and the persistence of life. Marylin and Mother, rocking in beds near one another, began to form a friendship, and then in mid-November Helen

Willie, another paralyzed mother of young children, joined the pair. I met Helen at the reunion that day in the Steputis backyard, and I gladly heard of the comfort the three women found in one another as they talked of their children and husbands, planned events at the center, and found solace in one another as women anywhere do.

December brought Mother's birthday, her twenty-ninth, and my fifth. Mother was feted at the center, and I suppose I was as well at my grandparents' house. For the Christmas holidays a garden club decorated the rooms and then on December 18, center graduates threw a party at the YMCA, and I was astounded to learn that Mother went. This was the first outing she'd had, other than to the airport to fly to Seattle, since falling ill in June, and I hungered to know what it meant to her. I like to think it did her good to be at such a festive occasion and in the midst of the strong and growing group of ex-patients, still struggling with their disabilities, but carrying on their lives. All she wrote in "The Vital Capacitor," however, was that she "had a delightful time." She further distanced herself by writing in the third person, saying that "Virginia represented the Center" at the "lovely Christmas party."

The staff and patients celebrated Christmas again on December 23 with refreshments and an exchange of gifts. The gifts, I assume, were purchased by volunteers and family at the direction of patients. Although all these holiday events were reported cheerfully by Mother in the newsletter, Christmas Day could not have been happy. No matter how much effort was made to make it pleasant, the day could not have been more unlike the Christmas a mother of two children might have hoped for. I think of the joyful celebrations I've had since becoming a mother, knee-deep in wrapping paper and well-being on Christmas morning, so confidently and gratefully a family, and I imagine my mother waking up that Christmas morning in 1954 on her rocking bed. I wonder whether she could even bear to think of what Kenny and I were doing that day, apart from her. Could she allow herself to wonder what the new year would bring?

MOST DAYS FELL TO WORK AND CARE that inched patients toward their goals of being the honored guest at a going-away party.

The daily routine started early, around 6:00 A.M., with sponge baths, toothbrushing, and dressing, followed by breakfast. For many patients, those simple morning tasks took considerable effort and help from staff members. Mother, among a few others, could do nothing for herself. Personal chores were out of the way by midmorning so that when the doctors made their rounds, the curtains that provided some privacy between beds could be opened.

The morning finished with occupational and physical therapy, followed by lunch at noon and a rest period until 1:30 P.M., when therapy resumed. For a quadriplegic, physical therapy consisted mainly of "passive range of motion" exercise. Damaged or destroyed muscles eventually became replaced with fibrous tissues that shortened and contracted. Those muscles had to be regularly stretched, "an extremely painful procedure which can be likened to the medieval torture known as 'the rack,'" recalled Arnold Beisser in his book *Flying without Wings*. Although polio patients often experienced extreme pain through physical therapy, the experience of the center's Elizabeth Wheelwright told her that if the body were kept supple, there should be no pain; loosening stiff muscles and joints was painful. She practiced the Sister Kenny method of muscle reeducation, working even with the muscles that appeared to have lost all function. With each patient, she and those she supervised went through each muscle group to create the motion the patients could not initiate on their own. She taught new patients anatomy, told them what the job of each muscle was, and spent whatever time it took to go over the entire body. Even patients who had no voluntary movement, like Mother, received physical therapy daily. "We didn't just assume nothing was there," Wheelwright told me, "or that nothing would come back."

Keeping joints and muscles supple is extremely important if a patient one day regains use of the muscles, but even patients who will never move those muscles again benefit from daily therapy. Without regular movement, the joints can become rigid and the body can draw into a fetal position, which makes care of the patient difficult and physical comfort almost impossible. Physiotherapy also helps prevent bed sores and relieves the pain that comes from staying in one position too long.

The patients at Harborview received physical therapy, which could take an hour, as much as six times a day, because the staff had seen that that's what it took to prevent stiffening. Everyone, including aides and orderlies, was taught techniques so that each patient was moved as much as possible. Family members were taught how to move fingers, arms, legs, and even trunk muscles so that if the patient went home for a night or weekend, they could keep up the treatments. And when family members came to visit, they were expected to pitch in. Plum always said, Wheelwright reported, that there was no need for anyone to just sit there visiting when they could be working the patient's fingers, arms, and elbows while talking. And he practiced what he preached. When making the rounds with student doctors, he paused at bedsides or wheelchairs and manipulated patients' fingers as he talked. Wheelwright recalls that when people came to observe, sometimes from other centers, they'd be amazed at how little trouble the patients had with stiffness. "It wasn't a problem," she says, "because we worked them so often." Dad learned the techniques and on his visits exercised Mother's fingers, hands, and arms especially. He said she was always grateful. "If you lay there long enough," he said, "you hurt everywhere."

Weekday mornings and afternoons at Harborview were also given to occupational therapy, with patients learning tasks that might contribute to a more independent life. Therapists searched for whatever usable motion a person had and capitalized on it. One teenager, paralyzed from the neck down, learned to write with a pen in her teeth, scratching out a page and a half in an hour of effort. One woman used her shoulder and trunk muscles to feed herself via a gadget with a spoon attached to a ball-bearing swivel. Patients with usable limbs learned to do everyday tasks at a "functional-activity board" equipped with latches, switches, and knobs where they practiced opening cabinets, turning dials, and moving levers. Those who could breathe for a time on their own exercised in the water therapy pool. A tilting bed helped patients who might walk one day begin to support their own weight in an erect position. With straps holding the patient against the bed, the patient stood on the footboard and rested her arms on a table-top. Therapists searched the patients' bodies for any working muscle, but many quadriplegics had only movements that were of little or no use, such as swaying a foot or wiggling fingers.

Nearly every day, in order to measure each patient's vital capacity or "V.C.," Dunning had patients blow into a tube, and the power of that air rotated a drum and created a precise graph. She often gave them more than one try to better their scores. Sometimes she used a fluoroscope to see what muscles the person used for breathing, another measure of progress. When a patient was being weaned to a new respirator or was ill, Dunning might take the measurement more than once a day as a simple monitor of how the patient fared. Carefully measured and heartily cheered, also, was the amount of time patients could breathe unassisted. Two minutes and twenty seconds for Shirley, fourteen minutes for Marylin, and for Virginia, a few breaths.

Each patient worked daily on his or her particular goals. Some recited poetry to increase vital capacity. One young boy exercised by riding a red tricycle around the wards. Others strengthened weak hands by molding clay. To increase her shoulder muscles, too weak to lift her arms, one woman learned weaving with her arms in slings, suspended from above, and the small loom sitting in her lap. Learning to shave oneself, write, or eat with or without slings was a big gain. Some patients could get in and out of bed alone and even remove their own shoes. Each item of progress was noted with fanfare in issues of "The Vital Capacitor." Helen put on her socks; Jeanne could untie her shoes; Jerry painted with a brush held by a mouthpiece; Hank shaved himself; Lauretta stood unassisted; Fred walked with crutches; John ate a bowl of Jell-o by himself; four patients increased their breathing time enough that they could go into the tub for water therapy. Shirley was labeled "a real gadabout" for her Sunday outings.

Elaine Easley, the fifteen-year-old girl who learned to write with her toes supported on a specially designed writing board, soon mastered algebra. After I heard of Elaine's accomplishment, I tried it myself, taping a pencil to my toes as I had seen done for her in a photograph. I could immediately write my name in big, wavering letters while leaning over my lap and concentrating on the shapes forming on the tablet below me. Looking again at a photograph of Elaine, I saw that she was rigid against a high-backed wheelchair, arms limp, respirator pumping, chin tucked, looking down the entire length of her body to the foot writing on a board below her. From there she did algebra and wrote letters. I read in "The Vital Capacitor" of these milestones and could not help but compare Mother's progress. She was learning to read with a machine that projected book pages onto the ceiling, using her mouth to turn the pages. As she waited out her first year of illness, she was still fully paralyzed, still fully dependent on machines for life.

The staff tried to teach Mother a technique called glossopharyngeal breathing, or frog breathing, for its gulping, jaw-flapping appearance. The technique, discovered by patients at Rancho Los Amigos Respirator Center at Hondo, California, enabled some respirator patients to be free of mechanical aids for hours at a time. It also gave patients like Mother, who had little capacity, a measure of safety should their respirators fail. Wheelwright traveled to Rancho Los Amigos to see the large operation there and learn how to teach the new breathing technique to her patients. The difficult procedure involved using the tongue to push air down the throat to the lungs (rather than swallowing gulps of air). Mother tried but couldn't master frog breathing. What held her back I'll never know. It was another hurdle she couldn't clear, another setback. And if all these years later, I feel let down, what must she have felt, trapped in a body that betrayed her daily?

IN ITS FIRST YEAR, twenty-two patients, including Mother, entered the center. All were severely crippled, and all, in the polio years before respirator centers, might have faced a future of complete invalidism. Most would have needed respirators for the rest of their lives. But that first year, twelve of the twenty-two were sent home. The majority of those twelve were breathing on their own most or all the time and were able to work, either as housewives or students, or at jobs outside their homes. But as 1954 came to a close, Mother was still there, with no plans being made to send her home. The only one who, I suppose, wasn't surprised by that was my father, who told me more times than I wanted to hear that he never had hope, never believed recovery was possible for her. And yet, while he was in Seattle, he wrote to a professor who was supposedly doing research with cobra venom as a cure for polio. He never received a reply.

Maybe when Dad saw there was no hope for full recovery, he saw no reason to hope at all. "I knew it was incurable, and she knew it, too," he said, thinking of those nightly visits in Seattle. "She was in misery. My heart was with her every minute." He then said something odd: "She died every time I left her at the hospital," meaning, I think, that he mourned her, though she still lived.

Each evening following dinner, which might be meat loaf, hot dogs, hash, or roast beef, patients prepared for visitors who came at 7:00 P.M. The women and girls made jokes in "The Vital Capacitor" about the bleakness of polio fashions. When other women of the time were wearing snug sweater sets with long straight skirts or full-skirted dresses pinched at the waist, pearls, and small hats, paralyzed patients were condemned to clothing that had to be roomy enough to wrap around the chest respirators and button down the front. Skirts often had no back (to prevent the discomfort of lying and sitting on wrinkles all day), a style that proved troublesome when the paralyzed female had to be lifted and moved. As for their hair, they had the do that inevitably came with lying with one's head always against a rest, the "polio poodle," also called the rooster tail. Hair formed either a halo or a topknot, instead of falling into whatever style a woman wished it might.

Mary Bready remembered that her hair was washed only once or twice in her three-month hospital stay when she was confined to bed. Such activities made for a disruption in hospital routine that the head nurse didn't like. "Gaining permission was such a belittling process," she remembered, "that it was hardly worth the while." Knowing that, I'm grateful to the people in Seattle who helped give my mother a measure of dignity with something so simple as curling her hair. I think of them and long to have done something for her myself. Often, when thinking of her, I'm the five-year-girl who wants to be mothered; but other times, I'm the forty-five-year-old me feeling maternal toward the twenty-nine-year-old Virginia who was in such great need. And then I'm a child again, fantasizing of magical power that would allow me to go back and undo what had been done to her.

WHEN DAD WENT IN THE EVENINGS, he and Mother had what he called "visits," chatting with each other and other patients and their families about the day. Dad scratched Mother's itches— "she would be so grateful," he recalls—and attended to her personal care by adjusting her position with propped pillows behind her back, bottom, and knees; by rolling her a bit to one side or the other; and by arranging her arms and fingers in various positions, as even slight shifts could bring comfort. "We'd try to carry on life with the visits," Dad says, "because that was our life." How each evening went, he told me, depended on Mother's condition. If she had a cold and wasn't feeling well or was upset about something, he tried to "smooth things over." If they could avoid it, they didn't talk about anything painful or difficult, mainly the future and us children, as that was sure to upset Mother. "She wanted so much to hold you kids in her arms," Dad told me, "and we talked about it once or twice, but it always made her cloud up, so I didn't want to press it." Dad couldn't remember whether Kenny and I wrote to Mother while she was in Seattle, a small fact that puzzled and worried me. Surely we wrote, surely my grandmother insisted on it, yet Dad didn't recall a single note or school paper or photograph sent from Colorado. Then, when I traveled to Seattle, Helen Willie told me that Mother did get mail from us—and it always made her cry. Helen also told me that Mother was learning to type with a wand in her mouth so she could write letters back.

Dad told me that during his visits, especially on Sundays, he often read the newspaper to Mother. I sat in the library and read those issues of the *Seattle Times* on microfilm and tried to imagine which of the articles he might have pointed out to her. Maybe the antics of Bobo, the new gorilla at the zoo, or such odd human-interest stories as one about twins born in the backseat of a car. But, for the most part, the news surely held little interest for her. With the exception of my father, everyone she knew in Seattle was with her every day at the hospital, so all the items about births, deaths, marriages, and social events of interest when reading a local newspaper held no intrigue. All she really wanted to see, Dad said, were the funnies, the adventures of the likes of Blondie and Dagwood, Dotty Dripple, Mutt and Jeff,

Mary Worth and Rex Morgan, M.D., Brenda Starr, Emmy Lou, Dick Tracy, and Moon Mullins.

Dad's nightly visits lasted, he remembers, two or three hours. The day ended with the task of getting all the patients settled for the night, which might include hooking them up to whatever breathing device they needed for sleep, caring for the tracheotomy hole, doing other routine night cleaning, and changing their clothing. Dad learned to suction Mother by sliding open the nickel-sized cover of her tracheotomy hole and running a rubber-tipped hose slowly into her tender throat to pull the phlegm out.

"I don't think I could have done a better job," is how Dad remembers his months there. He's told me that almost any time I've asked about the Seattle episode, insisting that Mother even told her mother that no one could have given her better care than he during that time. "Maurine told me she said it," Dad once wrote in a letter to me. He explained his good behavior by saying that maybe it was because he'd always been a "giver," having been as a toddler and young boy his ill father's "slave." Jesse Black, who had owned a car dealership before becoming ill even before my father, his seventh child, was born, is known to me only by his reputation for a fierce temper. Hearing Dad call himself a "giver" struck me as odd and ill-fitting. I interpret the term to mean someone who finds pleasure in caring for others, but I've always seen my father as a man with an insatiable need to be cared for. And it makes more sense to me that a four-year-old boy deprived of his father's care and made to serve would become a man still hungry for the solicitude he had deserved and missed as a child. From what I've learned, it appears that one good fit between my parents when they married was that Dad was needy and Mother liked to mother. She was, as her cousin Katherine Donald liked to say, always rooting for the underdog. And then polio ruptured that balance and left Dad in his young adulthood giving succor to his wife, whom he had come to rely on for emotional and physical needs. And it left her, who seemingly found meaning and reward in caring for him and her children, without purpose.

Dad tells me he made an effort to be cheerful at every visit, because if he wasn't, she'd become morose. All in all, he remembers, "she took it like a trooper." On both their parts, it seems, the good cheer was a facade for the benefit of the other. Dad's drinking began in earnest in Seattle as "a way to block things off," he told me. Only twenty-nine then, he was fit and his athletic body helped him hide the drinking. I suppose he mainly drank after leaving her at night, but he told me that at least one night he did his drinking before going to see Mother. On the way in, a nurse stopped him in the hallway. His listing walk and the alcohol on his breath made his condition obvious, and she sent him away, telling him, "You're in no shape to cheer anyone up. Go home and get some sleep." Dad says that was the only night he missed visiting Mother, but a friend of Mother's remembers that Dad sometimes telephoned to say he couldn't make it that night because he was in some other town on business. The town might be Bothell, within easy reach of downtown Seattle, but Mother didn't know the local geography. Alcohol provided a social life for Dad as well as an escape. He went out with some of the other husbands of patients for a drink and smuggled beer in for Archie Warnke, one of the patients there.

Perhaps alcohol helped him keep up the front of cheerfulness. Whatever efforts he was making, however, were set back when he got word in March that his mother, living in Boulder, was dying of cancer. He and his brother Roland, who lived in Oregon, drove to Colorado to her bedside. She was still conscious when they arrived, and in the brief conversation they had, she instructed my father: "Be nice to the kids." She went into a coma, and Dad and Roland drove back to the Northwest. A week later news came that she had died.

Surely when Dad and his brother visited their mother in Boulder, they came to see us children, too, though no one remembers it. I do, however, have a clear memory of Maurine, whom we lived with, drawing Kenny and me around her to tell us of Gramma Black's death. Sitting on a red vinyl padded stool at the breakfast bar, she told us the sad news. I sat on her lap, smelling the thick sweetness of the hoyas that grew from pots on either side of the window, vining up each side to meet at the top. In front of me, Kenny's turtle, Petey, sat in numb silence on a rock in the fishbowl that was his home. Gramma Black had given Kenny the turtle. She had once asked each of us what pet we wanted. He wanted a turtle and I wanted a horse, but knowing it was too much to ask for, I had said, "A kitten." I had, really, wanted a kitten, but for some reason she had not gotten me one. All I could think that day as I sat on Maurine's lap, looking at Petey and trying to picture what Gramma Black looked like now that she was "gone," was that I'd probably never have a kitten. I don't think I cried, but Kenny did. Until recently when my father set me straight, I had thought that memory came later, after my mother's death. Strong as the memory is, it has always had a stuporous quality. The visual details are clear, but the sense of what was being told to me was not. I see now that though my mother was not yet dead, her absence had led me into a daze. My five-year-old sensibility simply couldn't take in the complicated events that were coming down around me.

The accumulation of Dad's sorrows, beginning with his father's death when he was just four years old, must have driven him deeper into emotional debt. He had no one to confide in and would have seen seeking psychiatric help himself as a sign of weakness. Remembering those times, he wrote to me recently, "I was completely devastated and really alone—the outsider in every sense."

As for Mother, Dad remembers that although she had times of depression, she was usually cheerful. But Fred Plum and Marcelle Dunning remember Mother differently. "I worried about her," Plum told me, "because she never got over her depression. She cried a good deal of the time." Dunning remembers her as having such a difficult time emotionally that she asked the consulting psychiatrist to spend some extra time with Mother and get to know her for whatever aid he could offer. I asked Dunning if my mother was, as my father remembered, "the worst of the bunch." She answered carefully: "She may have had the worst trouble, if not the worst physical involvement."

Dad's only memory of Mother's time with the psychiatrist was finding Mother weeping one evening. That day the psychiatrist had confronted her with the question "How does it feel to know you'll never hold your children again?"

"I knew what he was trying to do," Dad told me. "He was trying to talk tough and make her face her situation." Dad's swagger as he tells this story is painful to me. He's told it repeatedly and each time emphasizes how he then talked tough back to the doctor and told him never to come around Mother again because if he did, Dad would break his legs. And that, according to Dad, was the end of Mother's psychiatric help. "I was a different guy then," Dad tells me now, remembering his temper and cockiness.

There's nothing about this story that I like. But for Dad to tell it differently, without its macho veneer, perhaps would open him to suffering he doesn't want to feel. Although I doubt a psychiatrist would allow a hollow threat to keep him from a patient in need, I wonder what kind of psychiatric help Mother did get in Seattle and how effective it was. At first I wanted to dismiss Dad's story altogether, but I've heard of other polio patients subjected to a confrontational style of psychotherapy, so perhaps it was part of the conventional thinking. Lou Sternburg told in his book of the psychiatrist coming to visit him three times a week and sitting on a high stool behind Lou in his iron lung. " 'How's your sex life, Louis?' " the doctor asked him. The husband of a woman rendered quadriplegic by polio told me that when she left a respirator center in the Midwest, they both had to get a psychiatric evaluation. Telling me about his interview, these forty years later, still made him angry. He wanted to punch the psychiatrist for asking him why he was sticking by his wife and taking care of her. "Are you hoping to get praise from others?" the doctor asked.

Surely Mother must have floundered, her life having become unrecognizable, her purpose and place lost, and nothing new to replace it. Where would she find the psychological strength to survive her circumstances? I wonder whether she experienced the same kinds of thoughts that Arnold Beisser described in *Flying without Wings*. "I had fantasies," he wrote, "or perhaps they were hallucinations, of a surgical procedure that would separate the head so that it would be unencumbered by the body. Perhaps it could be reattached to another body, or simply kept alive by a machine. Such ideas now seem bizarre, but they seemed quite reasonable in the light of the confused understanding I had about what was me and what was not, which was my private space and which belonged to someone else." As time went on with him in his paralyzed state, breathing with mechanical help, he came to long for something to die for. "I had recurrent fantasies of a suicide mission for some great, unspecified purpose," he wrote. "A thinking human being was required to carry it out, but physical ability was irrelevant. An honorable death seemed far better than the life I feared. But what an irony that I should need something to die for to make living worthwhile." I wonder what, in those weeks that turned to months in Seattle, Mother lived for. Beisser wrote of his battle with paralysis almost forty years after the fact. What conclusions could Mother have possibly come to in the first months of her durance? With no special intellectual gifts that I'm aware of, with little more than a conventional high school education, would Mother have found ideas rattling around in her head that would have given her suffering meaning? I wonder, and then I come back to my brother and me. I know that were I forcibly apart from my children, the prospect of reuniting with them would be reason enough to wait.

I KNOW LITTLE about what Kenny and I were doing in those months Mother was in Seattle, except that in September, Kenny enrolled in second grade and I in kindergarten at Sacred Heart of Jesus, a Catholic school where Benedictine nuns taught. I have many memories of the school, but none of them from kindergarten. I had a lay teacher that year, but all my classroom memories of that school involve the nuns. I have no memory, other than the death of Gramma Black, that I can tie to those months Mother was in Seattle. All I have are what others have told me. Maurine recalled for me a weekend drive in the mountains with Hayes driving and Kenny and me in the backseat. We were bumping along a dirt road when a storm gathered dark clouds above us. She asked Hayes to turn back, in hopes we could get out of the mountains before the rain broke. Probably hearing the anxiety in her voice and feeling the danger in an impending downpour, Kenny stood behind her and wrapped his arms around her neck, saying, "I'm glad we have a Mommy and Daddy to look after us until ours come back."

On Sunday afternoons Maurine and Hayes took Kenny and me with them to Denver to visit Maurine's parents, who lived next door to Maurine's Aunt Sarah and her daughter, Katherine, in matching brown row houses. Katherine remembers that one time, during those months we waited for Mother to come home, a friend came to visit Katherine while we were there. When she left, Kenny announced that he thought she was beautiful. When Katherine agreed, I reportedly put my hands on my hips in a gesture borrowed from my grandmother and said, "You don't think she's as pretty as Mommy, do you?"

There we were, two children who were told next to nothing, living with their grandparents, remembering a pretty mommy, and waiting for her to come back to us. For more than thirty years I gave that girl hardly a thought, though she lived within me, still waiting.

MOTHER SUFFERED SETBACKS, both emotional and physical, along the way in her rehabilitation. One incident that took a toll on her, according to Dad, was an outing to Helen Willie's house. Helen's brother sold cars and borrowed a station wagon off the lot to take Mother and Dad and Helen to the Willies' Seattle home for a Sunday afternoon visit. Helen, who was able to breathe unaided for a time and who was gaining strength in her upper body, had gone home for visits herself and invited Mother and Dad. Mother had already been out once, for the Christmas party, which apparently went smoothly enough for her to try again. This outing, however, was entirely unsuccessful. Mother was frightened throughout that she wouldn't be able to breathe. She rode in back of the station wagon, probably on a wheeled stretcher, with a battery-run respirator on her chest. The battery, which had a life of four or so hours, didn't pump with the strength of the respirators driven by electricity. And although Dad and a nurse accompanied her to deal with the wires and plugs, and the oxygen and suction equipment if needed, Mother couldn't relax.

Maybe this outing to a friend's house, to meet her children and see her home, was too close to the life Mother remembered and desired and yet too unlike the past for it to be tolerable. At the hospital and even at the Christmas party with former patients, disability was the norm. Perhaps this simple visit to a friend's house in a car was too severe a reminder of how far she had to go to get back into the world she had known. When they reached the Willies' house, she was too weary and frightened to endure being unloaded with her gear and wheeled into the house. The station wagon turned around to take her back to her rocking bed.

Lou Sternburg's first outing, also in a friend's station wagon, went a similar way. He had gone to his parents' house, accompanied by his wife, a nurse, and two aides. They got him in the house with difficulty, but when it came to getting him out, the stretcher knocked into doorways, wires were plugged in wrong, and he was in a panic. No one enjoyed the trip. When he got back to the safety of the hospital, he told a nurse, " 'That was awful,' " and said he wasn't going out again. She replied: " 'It's like falling off a horse. You have to get up and get on again. . . . You have to get away from this place where everyone's like you and out into the world.' " I don't know whether anyone said any such thing to Mother, but I do know she didn't go out again until she was discharged.

After being the sole adult respirator patient for most of her time in Phoenix, she now had others to compare herself to, and the comparisons would have been difficult to accept in two ways. Progress for patients as crippled as Mother often was heartbreakingly slow: a year spent learning to swallow for one bulbar patient, eighteen months for a quadriplegic to build up strength to breathe an hour or two alone. These were important, even essential, gains, yet they were so far from what many patients could do before polio that both the past and the future surely became, at times, unbearable to contemplate. Yet Mother had seen others who had been severely paralyzed recover muscle power. Her friend Marylin Angell, who had been devastatingly ill when she entered the Northwest Respirator Center in an iron lung in July 1954, two months before Mother, left in February 1955. She'd nearly died there and had given birth to her second son, and yet she was able to walk when she left. Her other special friend, Helen Willie, who had arrived in November, was also making good progress breathing on her own. Yet from what Dunning and others have told me, seeing how others were doing deflated Mother, rather than bolstered her. Watching others leave, even those much improved, could have been discouraging in another way. Although some people walked out or some who arrived in iron lungs left breathing on their own, no one was discharged restored to their prepolio condition. What was going on was helpful, but clearly it was not a cure.

Living with other severely handicapped people, Mother also had plenty of reminders of the fragility of her existence. Often a patient choked or a breathing machine failed. What next? Who next? Fears traveled through the rooms, according to a study done at the Mary MacArthur Unit in Boston, with illness in one patient mobilizing fears in all. "Stormy weather immediately aroused general concern about power failure, and the anxiety generated by one instance of mechanical difficulty with the respiratory equipment did not subside for several days," according to the researchers. Despite the cheerfulness of "The Vital Capacitor" reports, the same fears and anxieties circulated in the respirator rooms at Harborview.

The discharge of patients could be traumatic for those left behind. Researchers at the Mary MacArthur Respirator Unit noticed that discharges could reactivate patients' anxiety about their own homecomings and could set off disruptions in the surrogate family balance. They saw that when a forty-four-year-old patient, a "father figure" to the others, was released at the same time that a well-liked nurse left, several patients had severe reactions. Two women had to go back into tank respirators. A girl almost blacked out from inability to get a good breath, and another thought she was coming down with an infection. The timing of these incidents, the researchers said, was "highly suggestive."

Hospitalized in Baltimore with a severe case of polio, Norma Duchin developed a friendship with a woman who was at the hospital nine months with "weak-muscle polio," a case not nearly as devastating. When Duchin's new friend was discharged, walking, Duchin observed her departure by the mirror on her iron lung. "It was truly a moment of misery for me," Duchin wrote. "I had lost a friend, and I knew that I would never be leaving to step into an automobile." Similar emotions must have tortured Mother as she watched other patients, perhaps Marylin Angell in particular, go home. She gained and lost friends, and saw in their discharges the contrast with her own condition.

Although Mother's troubled emotional state could have come solely from her awareness of her condition, it may have had physical roots as well. An imbalance of oxygen and carbon dioxide in the circulatory and respiratory systems can change behavior, causing insomnia, restlessness, fatigue, anxiety, mental confusion, depression, and disorientation. The NFIP's Morton Seidenfeld, the director of psychological services and public education, reported to the 1954 national meeting that it was nearly impossible to separate the psychological from the physiological when such an imbalance occurred. He said that although there was a great deal of conflict and confusion about the emotional changes occurring in patients with breathing difficulties, there was "little doubt that such patients very frequently [underwent] serious alterations in their behavior, especially with regard to loss of emotional control."

MOTHER'S SETBACKS AND REMINDERS of her precarious physical condition were not only emotional but demonstrably medical. Two serious ones plagued her: high blood pressure and kidney stones. High blood pressure was common in the initial assault of bulbar polio, as the portion of the brain that controls automatic impulses, including blood pressure, could be profoundly disturbed. For most patients, however, passing through the crisis and receiving adequate ventilation put their blood pressure back in normal ranges. For a few, however, the blood pressure and cardiac irregularities continued beyond the crisis stage and could not be explained by inadequate ventilation. Mother was one of those. She arrived in Seattle with her blood pressure high, which the doctors thought could have come from her flight. But over time, it stayed high, despite efforts to control it with a low salt diet, carefully controlled ventilation, and counseling to reduce her fears.

She also had kidney stones, a concern that received research attention at the Northwest Respirator Center. Inactivity, in this case brought on by paralysis, can lead to demineralization of the bones, which releases calcium into the system and can result in ureter, bladder, and kidney stones. For polio patients, however, something more than inactivity was involved in the loss of calcium. The doctors didn't know why, but polio patients sometimes excreted as much as five or six times as much calcium as healthy people. They did know that despite those high amounts, they could, with careful management, prevent kidney stones. The deposits not only cause excruciating pain but can lead to infections, can require surgical correction, and can irreversibly damage the kidneys. Not a single patient who arrived at the Northwest Respirator Center without kidney stones developed them there, a point of pride for the staff. "Our whole effort was prevention," says Dunning, "because there was not much we could do once a patient developed them." Mother, however, arrived with kidney stones, which compromised both her immediate and her long-term health. While there, she had surgery to remove them, heaping yet more onto what she had to endure.

"A large urinary output," as one resident physician put it, was the most important single factor in preventing kidney stones. Each patient had to consume at least three quarts of liquid each day, which was carefully measured and monitored, as was every "output," which was expected to be two quarts daily. Every day each person's urine was collected in a jug, then measured and analyzed by the lab technician for its calcium concentration. (What Archie Warnke's unauthorized beer consumption did to those careful measurements is anyone's guess.) For people with swallowing difficulty or labored respiration, drinking three quarts of liquid each day could take a big effort, especially when the staff was also encouraging them to eat. Patients' diets were carefully monitored also, to ensure that they had a low-calcium diet.

Most of the patients had trouble with constipation, and so part of the daily routine was the dispensing of drops of stool softener. The amount of food each person ate each day and the volume of each stool were also measured. All that attention to bladders and bowels, however necessary, only added to the lack of privacy for paralyzed polio patients. Lou Sternburg once had to move his bowels while being transferred from his rocking bed to a tub, and rather than take the time to put him back in bed with a bedpan, the three aids stood over him while he used it. "With all the losses I had suffered—breathing, movement, freedom—the worst blow to my pride was the loss of privacy," he wrote, remembering that incident. For patients who had limited or no mobility, maintaining privacy about bodily matters was impossible. Women even had to allow someone else to put on and change their menstrual pads. At best, patients lost self-consciousness and failed to be embarrassed with the help of staff who could laugh and joke with them about the predicament. As the wife of a quadriplegic said, "There's no way someone who has to pee in a bedpan for the rest of his life or who has a hole in his throat from which stuff bubbles and oozes can function unless he is eased toward it." Dunning, like other physicians for respirator patients, viewed the openness of the wards as an aid in helping patients accept their situations.

Lost privacy was measured in other ways, too. Janet Steputis said that when her husband, Hank, was moved to the Northwest Respirator Center from the hospital, they both missed the private time they'd had together in his hospital room. In the center, her husband lived in the open room with others, having only the privacy that came from a drawn curtain around his bed. The trade-off was the socializing and support received from the other patients and families. For Mother, I suspect it was an easy trade: the loneliness of the Phoenix hospital for the bustle of the staff in Seattle and the friendship among the patients.

THE SUMMER I VISITED SEATTLE and met many of the people who had been there with Mother, I asked Bertha Doremus about her social-work assessment of patients. As I sat down next to her, in the filtered sun of Janet Steputis's backyard, I hoped that she could tell me what I really wanted to know. As important as the medical information was, what I wanted to hear was how Mother fared emotionally. Doremus, however, remembered little specifically about my mother, but carefully explained in detail how she evaluated patients' circumstances and what kind of help she could offer.

She looked first to the patients' roles and how polio had affected them. She remembered talking to one paralyzed mother, not mine, though I feel sure it could have been, who said, "I'm no good as a mother now." Doremus replied: "Who else could be a mother to your children? Your husband could remarry, but no one could replace you as mother." She also looked to the basic relationships, usually family relationships, that might provide strength to the patient. She looked for other resources that might support the patient, such as housing, finances, and connections to community and church or other groups.

And finally, she looked at the person's reaction to the illness and disability, which often was a tangled emotional bramble. When someone suggested to Elaine Easley, the teenage girl whose arms were lost to paralysis, that she learn to write with her feet, she completely dismissed the idea as being ridiculous, wrong, not normal, not fitting with her idea of herself. But eventually the staff penetrated her resistance and the girl learned to write. Doremus, working with the entire staff and family, tried to help each patient deal with his or her individual trouble areas.

I listened to all this that August day in 1994, struggling to keep my face from showing the torment I felt. There I was that day, meeting and talking with people who had lived and worked with my mother, wanting to hear every detail of what they remembered of those times, and yet too often I asked a question and got an answer I didn't want to hear. What Bertha Doremus had to say only confirmed that in every possible way Mother was at a deficit. Her roles in life were all familial, and had she remained in her severely crippled condition, an adaptation to being mother, wife, and daughter would have been extreme. She had no other work that might bring her satisfaction or a sense of purpose. And I wondered how much strength she could have received from her family relationships. For her first two months in Seattle she had no family or friends nearby, and then only Dad. And what other resources did she have? She had religion, Catholicism, but no church. She had a hometown, but whatever community she had had there drifted away in the years she spent in Oregon and Arizona. She had no house of her own where her two children and husband waited for her return. And her reaction to her illness was, as best I can glean, fraught with fear, discouragement, and depression.

THEN, FOR REASONS I DON'T KNOW, sometime in the spring of 1955, Mother's outlook began to change. Dunning told me that she began to face the fact that the little bit of progress she had made was all that she would get. I wonder whether simply the passage of time and the association with other people who shared her experiences finally began to change her. Reading the newsletter from the Seattle unit, I could see how important the activities of those who had been discharged were to those still confined. The newsletter contained detailed descriptions by ex-patients of new and adapted equipment, such as wheelchairs, lifts, respirators, and even chair cushions and where to buy them. The newsletter told how they coped and what they accomplished. One teenager wrote an account of how, during her first day out of the hospital, she realized that no nurse was around to finish feeding her her meals, and so she devised a "scheme and as a result . . . [had] fed [herself] completely ever since."

Whatever the catalyst, Mother finally began, as Dunning told me, "to see that life was a possibility." She finally "could visualize being in a rocking bed at home." And as soon as the staff saw that, they began to make plans to send her to Colorado. Their decision to send her home couldn't have been one that sent great cheer through the staff. They knew she was being discharged with continuing serious problems. She was still completely paralyzed, still had kidney trouble, and still had to be deeply reclined in a wheelchair in order to breathe on a portable respirator. She could not breathe on her own enough to survive a power outage longer than a breath or two. She still needed a tracheotomy, further complicating home care. "We knew her problems were severe," Dunning said, "and we didn't know what was going to happen to her or how long she would survive." But ultimately the staff thought she'd be better off at home with her family. Mother had, in the parlance of the respirator centers, "received maximum predictable benefit."

Patients stayed, according to its policies, until they had a home service developed to provide ongoing personal, respiratory, and medical care, as well as ongoing rehabilitation to the previous job or other rehabilitation goal. The process for discharge included "at least" one visit to the person's home, according to Doremus, who was the key individual in preparing a patient to go home. She made home visits not only to Washington State residents but also to people in Idaho and

Oregon, and even to some at a remote Blackfoot reservation in Montana and to Anchorage. She went to "evaluate and interpret home-care needs, especially for accessibility in the home for the wheelchair, rocking bed, bathing, and toileting." She went to see whatever work the person might do and to check on transportation to a physical therapist, occupational therapist, and physician. Doremus made an effort to interpret whatever needs the patient had to the family, as well as to local support people, the various therapists, and a physician. The staff developed a form for the family members to fill out regarding the physical layout of the house, including the width of doorways to see whether a wheelchair could pass through. They also made sure there was back-up power in the case of electrical failure and a wheelchair ramp for getting out of the house. In her travels to a patient's community, paid for by the NFIP, Doremus visited the local hospital to see whether it was set up to handle an emergency with a respirator patient. She talked to family members to make certain they were ready for the patient and wanted the patient at home.

Whenever possible, patients went home for short overnight stays before discharge in order to give both the family and the patient practice at the procedures and to ease anxiety. If the family lived too far away for overnight visits, they were encouraged to come a few days before discharge to learn techniques of nursing care, such as how to suction, as well as some physiotherapy and information about the patient's machinery.

Mother was discharged without such a detailed plan, however, since Colorado was outside the range of Doremus's travels. Likely arrangements were made by mail and telephone with a physician and a social worker in Boulder and with the local March of Dimes. But no one counseled my grandparents about her return or taught them how to care for her. Perhaps they didn't even know that my grandmother would become Mother's primary caregiver.

SOMETIME IN THE LATE SPRING OF 1955, arrangements were made for the NFIP Seattle chapter to fly Mother home, and the Boulder chapter to greet her. The date of her departure remained uncertain for weeks, pending some final details I couldn't pinpoint, perhaps the availability of an airplane. Once the day was settled, however, the staff and patients threw a going-away party for Mother, and a reporter and a photographer from the *Seattle Times* visited the hospital to record her departure. The article, with a headline "POLIO PATIENT TO REJOIN CHILDREN," quoted Mother as saying, "We were just preparing to move from Phoenix back to Boulder, Colo., where I was born and raised, when polio struck. Now, at last, I can go home again. I can see my children again." The reporter noted that her "constant companion" would be the portable electric respirator and that she would go home to "begin an unfamiliar life in a familiar setting."

Again, I sat staring at a grainy newspaper photograph, searching for my mother. That one shows her smiling as she sits in a high-backed wheelchair, with a hose that connects the shell covering her chest to a metal table on wheels, which holds her battery respirator and suctioning machine. She looks wooden, like a string puppet. Her arms, from shoulder to wrist, are uniformly thin, without the slightest flab or muscle definition. Her hands lie in her lap. Her skinny legs and swollen ankles, covered with white stockings, rest unnaturally on the footrests of her chair. Whoever placed her feet, in their unfashionable lace-up shoes, left one askew, giving her a knock-kneed appearance. She's wearing a skirt, but seems to have nothing on her upper body except that shell. Something I can't make out in the old newsprint copy I have, given to me by the nurse Shirley Chiles, sits on Mother's right shoulder. I think it might be a corsage.

Mother made this trip, again in a specially arranged C-47, in a wheelchair rather than an iron lung. Once again she traveled alone, with Dad following later in the car. Mother left on Saturday, June 11, 1955, ending the second major stage in her polio care. Next, she would try to resume a life with her children and husband. I'm convinced that she wanted desperately to go home, that she wanted to see her parents and, most of all, Kenny and me. But I can't help wondering what other thoughts went through her mind as she made this second unusual airplane journey. Did she leave her friends and the staff reluctantly? Did she wonder whether she would get the kind of medical and personal care she needed at home? Did she know who would provide the care? Did she know enough about what might be coming for her and our family in Boulder to be afraid? What did she think when she looked out the window overlooking the Seattle seaport for the last time, saying goodbye to Oscar, the seagull, whom she called "one of the most faithful and popular callers at the Center"?

CHAPTER SIX

Weathering Reality

As I learned more and more, it became clear to me that, in my mother's story and in those of other victims, the considerable physical repercussions polio often left were intimately tangled with social and psychological complications and considerations. Leonard Kriegel, who lost the use of his legs to polio at age eleven, wrote: "While the consequences of polio were primarily physical—I would never again be able to walk without braces running the full length of my legs, and crutches in my hands—my disease had profound nonphysical ramifications from the beginning." In my search for what those additional consequences were in the lives of victims and their families, I found a great deal of help in the 1987 book *Stories of Sickness*, by the physician Howard Brody. The author did not specifically address polio, but clearly his ideas apply. Brody looked at the dual nature of illness—"the way it can make us different persons while we still remain the same person"—and how that affects a person's life and self-image. While those polio-changed bodies contained the self that had existed before the disease, the new physical limitations demanded something different, something more, from the individual. In Brody's theory, disease has profound nonphysical results because it forces one to rewrite one's life story. "We are, in an important sense," he said, "the stories of our lives. How sickness affects us depends on how sickness alters those stories."

What revisions polio would demand in a life narrative depended to a significant degree on the extent of the residual paralysis, but also, I found, on personality, expectations, age, life experiences, and circumstances. While I was delving deeper and deeper into my mother's experience, and finding there a dark tale of suffering, through the stories of others I was repeatedly reminded of the infinite range of experiences polio covered.

Reading Mary Bready's unpublished memoirs, I was struck by her cheerfulness and resilience throughout three months in a hospital and, once discharged, during the time of learning to walk without a brace. Polio dominated a period in her life, but it was an episode, and not an unusually sad or defining one at that. That was partly so, I suspect, because before the disease found her, she had both an attitude and a family that provided strength and structure. She and her husband had the same, unspoken thought on the day she was taken to the hospital, which was that they "were facing a new adventure, a new challenge to be met and defeated." And then the disease cooperated in fulfilling their expectations. It didn't present more than they could incorporate into their ongoing life scheme. Polio affected only one leg, and not too severely. Once out of the hospital, Mary's life could, for the most part, pick up where it left off. Yet even as I write the words *only one leg*, I imagine the child left with "only one leg" slightly damaged who might go on to ride a bike and roller-skate and dance, but never with the ease and naturalness of his or her playmates, the child who might have gained with the disease a never-to-be-shaken sense of being among those on whom misfortune falls. The experience of polio, I found again and again, did not yield to easy generalizations.

The severity of crippling wasn't the only factor in how this disease affected a life. How people experienced it and how much psychological suffering it brought didn't go lockstep with physical effects, measured along a line of emotional misery, from full recovery at one end to respiratory quadriplegic at the other. One weakened limb didn't exact some precise, predictable amount of psychic suffering. No one can measure, for example, what it has meant to a mother of eight children, who fell ill when her sixth child was in the womb, not to have hugged any of them again, and none of those born after her illness, because of the weakness in her upper body. "Oh," she said to me recently, "just to put your arms around somebody—it's a kind of ache." Who can measure the often subtle and tedious deprivations of a fettered life?

Children, even those who came through their polio experience without residual paralysis, suffered emotionally because of the trauma of hospitalization and abrupt separation from their families and normal activities. Researchers at the Pediatric Department of Harvard Medical School and the Children's Hospital of Boston followed fifty-two children with polio from 1943 through 1946 and searched for psychological aspects of the illness. They found that although many of the children in the study improved physically, they got worse in other ways. Even patients who made complete recoveries were "likely to be emotionally fragile and often showed psychological symptoms suggesting cerebral involvement. These difficulties combined with the emotional upheaval created by the illness resulted in many problems." During the first weeks following discharge, those children, for example, were "hyperactive, irritable, or disobedient, or, in some instances, too dependent or 'whiny.' " Children who required prolonged hospitalization and orthopedic care showed various disturbances, depending in part on their ages. Those between one and five suffered a lag in speech development in the first years of hospitalization (as they probably would have, had they been institutionalized for any other reason). Older children showed difficulty with concentration and general emotional fragility, especially in the first year, though "traces were still discernible for several years."

Surviving the crisis didn't immediately end the difficulties, as the family of J. Carlton Babbs, a Methodist minister in Cincinnati, learned. Mary, the youngest child, and only girl, of Carlton and Harriet Babbs had a high fever in 1952. When the doctor saw her neck stiffening, he ordered her to a hospital, where a spinal tap confirmed polio. Lying in a crib, Mary was lethargic, fevered, and unable to swallow any liquids for four days. At the end of that time, Mary's fever abated, and she resumed normal swallowing and breathing. The hospital released her, and her family joyfully welcomed her home. But the ordeal wasn't over yet. Mary, who seemed physically fine, save for paralysis on the left side of her face, wept continually, fussing through the days and keeping the family awake at night. Her parents understood that the reaction was expected, given the nature of the disease and the time of separation from the family, but they had no way to explain the trouble to her. Parents of other children who had had polio told them to expect this emotional disturbance to last as long as six months.

IN TRYING TO INTEGRATE the experience of polio, survivors often faced conflicts imposed by the nature of their disabilities, by their desires and limitations, and by the expectations of others. Integrating the experience meant incorporating it into one's life plan, according to Brody. The *life plan*, as he uses the term, refers to a view of one's life that is affirmed by close associates (such as friends and family) and that is rational, meaning it takes into account one's limitations and talents. Before polio, my mother's life plan, for example, was probably nothing more complicated than an expectation that she would graduate from high school, get married, have children and rear them, and eventually become a grandmother.

One way people cope with illness, one possible "story of sickness" as delineated by Brody, is to view it "as a lacuna in the narrative of one's life." The victim simply resumes life as if nothing happened, which, of course, is best suited to an acute illness rather than a chronic one. Some polio victims, like Mary Bready, were able to continue their life plans despite the interruption of polio because its residual effects allowed that. Released from the hospital and back at home in the large, aging house she and her husband had bought just before her illness, Bready found that in her leg brace she could still paint, hang wallpaper, sew, and garden, if a bit awkwardly. After wearing her brace for about two years, it broke and she took it to the brace shop at the hospital for repairs. Hearing that it would take three weeks, she decided on her own to get along without it rather than go back to crutches. "I walked in brightly to pick it up," she wrote, "and never put it on again; it is in the attic now as a reminder of how lucky I have been since."

For someone with greater paralysis to view an illness as an interlude rather than the main event, however, requires, as Brody says, "denying the severity of the disease, even if one does not deny the disease itself." I might have thought that was impossible for someone severely handicapped from polio had I not met Janet Steputis and her daughter, Chancy Grace, when I traveled to Seattle in the summer of 1994. Hank Steputis, who came down with polio in 1953 and was treated at the Northwest Respirator Center, could breathe about eight hours a day using his neck muscles (the strap muscles used to gasp in air). He rested and slept on a rocking bed. He had the use of his forearms and hands (although he couldn't use his thumbs). Despite his disabilities, he resumed his role as the family's breadwinner, starting with telephone sales from home, while his wife tended their two children. "We worked hard at having a normal life," Janet said. Her daughter, born four years after Hank became ill, told me: "The reality was that we weren't normal. But at school I could pass for normal." For the nearly thirty years that Hank lived after his encounter with polio, the Steputis family did its best to keep a cheerful outlook, to love one another, to live in the larger community of church and civic activity, to be "normal." And, as best I could tell, they succeeded by refusing to accept the dictates of polio. They could not deny Hank's handicaps, but they could deny what it meant in their lives.

Another story of sickness described by Brody that applies to many, perhaps most, polio survivors is one that "forces a modification of one's life plan." The new story of one's life includes the previous life plan up until the sickness occurs, "followed by a reexamination and a formulation of a new life plan that is rational given the limitations the chronic sickness is expected to impose." While one is formulating a new life plan, the old one must be grieved, because, as Brody wrote, the "old life, after all, was a major part of oneself, upon which all of one's claim to self-respect was based; one does not lightly undergo its loss."

What he had to say helped me greatly in understanding what my mother faced in her helplessness. "In extreme cases," Brody wrote, "one might even be justified in asserting that the old life plan was such a major part of oneself that to lose it is to lose one's identity, so that the only story that could be told of existence after the sickness is the story of the life of a different individual entirely." My mother lost herself to polio and, I think, floundered in her effort to replace her old identity, her old story, with a new one she could imagine living. The way the Steputis family coped by normalizing their life surely went a long way toward helping Hank maintain his personal integrity. Although desperately handicapped, he continued to participate in his family and community. As best I can tell from the stories Janet Steputis and Chancy Grace told me, Janet created, from the beginning of Hank's illness, a vortex that held Hank and the rest of the family together. She, along with her husband, I assume, were determined not to let polio force them to completely rewrite their future. My image of my mother, however, during those months in Phoenix and then Seattle is that she was alone, spinning in space, as was each of us in our family. She had been completely thrown off her place in the world.

Polio did not need to deal out such profound disabilities as my mother's to require considerable modification of one's life plans, however. "Until I met up with my virus," Leonard Kriegel wrote, "I was a monotonously average eleven-year-old boy," but thereafter, "I was no longer 'normal.'" Polio forced him to leave behind the boy he had been for eleven years and become someone else. "By the age of nineteen, I was already beginning to understand that no one ever 'conquers' disease and no one ever 'overcomes' its legacy. And yet I managed to look upon resistance to what my virus had made of me as the very essence of who I was as a person."

Some people, unable to forge an acceptable new identity out of the old, fought the changes. One woman told me that her mother, who was almost as crippled as my mother, resented efforts at rehabilitation. She hated the projects she was "put through" and despised the idea of "handicapped crafts." She hated the rocking bed and raged when her daughter, asked to draw a picture of her mother at school, drew her mother in a wheelchair. Perhaps, unable to do what she expected of herself, without breath and fingers and mobility, she refused the major revision her illness required.

THE STORIES OF SICKNESS that polio victims had to tell were affected, in part, by the public image of the disease. Whether polio altered, interrupted, or ruined a life, it invariably, at least temporarily, set the patient and family apart from the community in two ways. On one hand, victims and their families were quarantined and shunned; on the other, they were held out as celebrities.

Often the first separation was literal, through hospital isolation and quarantine, practices firmly established during the 1916 polio epidemic. That year, New York City, the center of the epidemic, saw 8,900 cases and 2,400 deaths between June and December. That was a mortality rate of one afflicted child in four. The besieged city went so far as to require people under age sixteen to produce a certificate showing that their homes were free of polio before they could leave the city. Police stood at highways and railroad stations to halt the exodus of thousands of city dwellers. Other municipalities employed the same measures. A certificate required for train travel out of Baltimore County, Maryland, dated September 1, 1916, indicated that as of 2:20 P.M., Captain F. B. Downing, age thirty-three and living in Pikesville, Maryland, and members of his family—his wife, age twenty-seven, and F. C. Downing, their nine-month-old son—were "in good health, [had] not had polomyelitis [*sic*] and [had] not been exposed to the same." It was signed by a health officer in Pikesville. (Ironically and sadly, F. C. Downing died forty years later in an iron lung, less than a month after getting polio. Had he been exposed to polio during that epidemic as an infant, he might have acquired a lifelong immunity to the disease.)

When a ten-year-old girl summering with her family in Maine in 1924 came down with a serious case of infantile paralysis, her parents wanted to take her home to Connecticut. But the three states she had to travel through, Maine, New Hampshire, and Massachusetts, each had different quarantine periods, with New Hampshire's being the longest. Once enough time had passed for the girl to travel from the other states, her parents obtained permission from New Hampshire to allow them to take the girl, secluded in a railroad cabin, through the state. As the southbound train hit the New Hampshire–Maine border, it made an unscheduled stop. New Hampshire health authorities stepped on, demanding to know where the girl was. When they found her, they sealed the door and windows of the cabin with brown tape, got off the train, and waved it on. When the train reached the New

Hampshire–Massachusetts state line, it stopped again. New Hampshire authorities there, after checking to make sure the tape had not been disturbed, sliced it open with a knife and sent the train on.

By the forties it was known that such measures were useless in controlling epidemics because much of the spread of polio came from those with inapparent or mild infections. Still, quarantines persisted. Sometimes families not directly touched by polio experienced the disruption of isolation. When the two older children in a Passaic, New Jersey, family were exposed to polio at a summer camp, an uncle was dispatched immediately to retrieve them. When they pulled up to their home, the children saw their father waiting on the street, his eyes full of suffering as he explained that the children couldn't see their younger brother and sister or their mother. They were being sent, instead, to the home of an aunt whose children were grown, where they would stay for weeks. "I remember a routine of carrot juice and daily baths and unutterable loneliness," said the daughter.

In 1949 attendees at a national conference on polio, along with other medical authorities, called quarantine regulation unwarranted and suggested a week or the duration of the patient's fever as the maximum hospital isolation. Quarantine and hospital isolation could create fear and hysteria during an epidemic and could prevent the patient from getting necessary treatment in the early stages, the health authorities said. And yet quarantines went on, dictated by law in some communities. Singling out and restricting polio's victims was the only way the public and some health authorities knew to deal with the disease.

Once health authorities removed a quarantine sign from a door, neighbors, friends, and even relatives weren't necessarily comfortable visiting. The fear of polio was so great and the association between "dirt and disease," as Naomi Rogers's book of that name argues, was so strong that cleansing rituals—for example, disinfecting the clothing and possessions of the ill or dead and confiscating the possessions patients took into isolation wards—were carried on without any evidence of their effectiveness. The actor Mia Farrow, who contracted polio at age nine, was the only one of the seven children in her family to get the disease. While she was hospitalized, her family gave away the dog, drained the swimming pool, reseeded the lawn, repainted the whole house, reupholstered the couch, and cleaned the carpets.

The line between quarantine and shunning muddled because the public carried sometimes conflicting attitudes toward polio. While the nation expressed its collective concern, notably through continued contributions to the March of Dimes, they also feared those who had polio. When Tex Blumenstock, a farmer who contracted polio at age thirty-eight, was hospitalized, his family was ostracized by all but a few friends and family members. Some people didn't want his children in school with theirs. Publicly, however, victims weren't blamed for their malady, as AIDS or even cancer and heart disease patients are today, because polio was difficult to tie to specific behavior. Instead of being seen as punishment for wrongdoing, it was seen as evil itself, which had to be conquered—a view that helped fuel the passionate and consistent giving.

Yet the crippling and pain of individuals suffering from polio repelled those who escaped its arbitrary slings. Although people resisted blaming polio on its victims—who could hold schoolchildren accountable for their braces and crutches or iron lungs?—many people wanted to believe that *something*, some mistake, misbehavior, or characteristic, distinguished the stricken from the hearty. For many people, believing that only luck divided them not only was too frightening but also conflicted with their psychological or religious beliefs.

As human beings, we search for cause and effect in the face of disaster and therein find comfort. God is often credited or blamed. The family of one severely paralyzed teenage girl heard through rumors that some people in the community thought the tragedy would never have befallen the girl if her parents had been churchgoers. The spared, it seems, want to see in the stricken evidence of justice served, to find meaning and purpose in random disasters, because then they can believe they are safe.

Leonard Kriegel described his mother's heartache when the butcher's wife announced that his illness was God's punishment of his mother. "Mad or sane," he wrote much later, "the butcher's wife had touched my mother's center. . . . For she had voiced precisely what my mother herself believed about disease in her own fear-ravaged heart. . . . Accident, illness, war, famine, disease: punishments visited upon one by the master of the universe." As Kriegel pointed out, the views expressed by that half-crazed, superstitious woman and his own "judgment-obsessed mother" decades ago are shared even today by "far more sophisticated and rational people. . . . To be a 'victim of disease' is to be tested, tried, made better, punished, reborn."

The need to explain and rationalize the irrational led both the public and polio survivors to assign meaning to the randomness of the disease. For the survivor, Kriegel wrote, it becomes increasingly difficult, as one focuses on the loss, "not to read into it some greater significance than it merits. . . . Physician and theologian join hands in assigning responsibility. Disease has somehow been welcomed, accident has somehow been sought out." And yet, he continued, this effort to "authenticate suffering" is a "grinding obscenity." Speaking for everyone touched by polio, he wrote: "I was not responsible for the chance encounter that allowed the virus to slip into my bloodstream in the summer of 1944. Punishment has nothing to do with the crime—unless the crime is defined as merely being human."

Many patients felt the assignment of blame as guilt, a common response to polio. Reporting on a study of children with polio, researchers wrote in the *New England Journal of Medicine*: "It is as if the patient thinks in such direct and elemental terms as these: a terrible thing has happened to me—I must have done something terrible to make it happen." Children in that study, done by the University of Maryland School of Medicine Psychiatric Institute, explained their polio by saying they ran around too much or played too much; one said he "wore his legs out" by riding his bicycle. Such feelings of responsibility seemed to account for the almost universal cooperation with the sometimes strict confinement; it was as if the children's restriction allowed them to atone for wrongdoing.

STILL, PARADOXICALLY, while this cheerless drama of guilt and blame was played out on one level, polio was the country's cause célèbre on another level. While some victims were shunned, others were set apart with extra attention, even a kind of celebrity. Given the extensive publicity, few could fail to be moved by the plight of polio victims. People eagerly read accounts like the story in *Coronet* magazine about the courage of the citizens of Hickory, North Carolina, a town that faced an epidemic in June 1944.

Polio raced through the rural area surrounding the quiet town of 13,487, but the nearest hospital, in Charlotte, was sixty miles away and so crowded that army tents set up on the hospital lawn served as an isolation ward. Faced with a growing population of polio cases and no way to care for them, the townspeople of Hickory set their minds to building their own hospital. In less than three days, they built and equipped a fifty-five-bed hospital with donated materials and labor. But the epidemic kept pace, and soon 224 cases were reported and 194 children crowded the hospital. Everyone pitched in. A lawyer whose son was hospitalized with bulbar polio worked in the hospital kitchen scrubbing the floors. Women of the town went house to house borrowing blankets and beds and soliciting nursing help. Help moved in from around the country in the form of doctors, nurses, specialists, physical therapists, supplies, and equipment to the improvised hospital. Giant army tents were erected there, too, to house the growing number of patients.

From June 1 to September 27, normal life stopped for the town as the people devoted themselves to building, in the next four months, an eight-structure hospital. The town donated $34,000 in cash and well over $50,000 in labor and material. In all, over four hundred patients were cared for, only six from the town itself. One polio specialist who had gone to the town to help said of the townspeople, "They have wrought a miracle."

Although few communities were faced with the extreme situation of Hickory, all around the nation neighbors and friends, like those of the Babbses's in Cincinnati, carried food to the porches of families sequestered behind quarantine signs. They raised money to build a room where a quadriplegic father could live at home. An ambulance service volunteered its equipment to transport a severely crippled man home for weekends. Neighborhood children entertained the homebound. Schoolteachers used their own time to help their ill students keep up while convalescing. Women's service groups took on local polio wards as projects. A teen club used the money from its treasury to take a teen polio patient to a movie.

At least for a short time, schoolmates often showed deference to their fallen peers. An entire elementary class might, for instance, visit a classmate in an iron lung or create get-well notes for a hospitalized pupil. In the summer before his senior year of high school, Dennis Samson contracted polio and spent a year out of school, hospitalized and convalescing. While he was away, his classmates voted him their first student of the month. It was "an honor," he noted, "I would have been unlikely to receive under ordinary circumstances." A local reporter did a story on him for the newspaper, and at the annual school Christmas pageant the choir sang him a personalized "We Wish You a Merry Christmas." He found that all the attention "mitigated my general condition to a degree."

Because the disease stayed so much in the front of public awareness, wards of polio patients, especially children, drew special attention of a wide sort. That was the case at the University of Michigan Hospital where Ruth Hazen worked as a nurse in 1948. Televisions were scarce in those days, but patients in the contagion unit had a few available and would gather around them to watch wrestling broadcasts, which were made even more attractive when a wrestling star from Detroit visited the unit one day. Hazen watched the celebrity go room to room, shaking hands and telling the patients he, too, had had polio, but had fully recovered. He also announced that that evening he was going to have a bout with a most disagreeable opponent, and he wanted the children to root for him, as that would surely help him win. His entourage arranged to supply each room with a TV, and the wrestler persuaded the head nurse to allow even the youngest patient, a four-year-old, to stay up to watch.

Hazen, off duty by the time of the bout, searched out a bar with a television set tuned to the match and settled in to watch. The announcer introduced the two wrestlers, saying the one had spent part of the day at the hospital, and the polio patients were all watching and cheering. In the arena and on the ward, as Hazen later learned, the disagreeable opponent was soundly booed, and from the outset there was little doubt about the outcome of the match. At the end, the defeated opponent sent his best wishes to the polio patients and assured everyone he had not hurt their hero.

Individually, too, children on polio wards sometimes received considerable special attention, which could make their stays pleasurable. Lynda D. W. Bogel recalled that when she was nine, she spent one miserable week hospitalized in fever, delirium, and pain; but when the week ended, she was sent to the general polio ward for a week's recuperation, which she "adored." "I had an entrancing, long-suffering, and friendly roommate, a very wealthy little blond ten-year-old," she wrote. The wealthy girl had every model of Ginny doll and steamer trunks full of clothes for them. The girls lay on their beds changing the dolls' costumes when they weren't learning how to knit, racing their wheelchairs, or having pool therapy. At night nurses slipped in to give them oranges. "Why these had to be snuck eludes me," she said, "maybe just to let us feel special." She had such a fine time that when her parents came to fetch her home, she cried in protest.

Fred Davis found among the families he studied that hospitalization "raised delicate and precarious issues." Children were expected "somehow to demonstrate an emotionally appropriate division of loyalties and attachments between home and hospital." Several of the children in his study were reluctant to go home, often saying they wanted to stay for upcoming parties or other entertainment planned for holidays. One twelve-year-old girl defiantly said that she could have much more fun in the hospital at Christmas than she could at home, and that she didn't want to leave before then. A seven-year-old boy, whose family was the poorest of those in Davis's study, "virtually had to be dragged away from the hospital, and for days thereafter he cried incessantly and insisted that he wanted to return."

In their efforts to help their children strike the right balance between home and hospital, some parents went a little too far, as illustrated by one mother who told Davis that she and her husband had spoken at length with their eight-year-old son about how important it was for him to learn to like the hospital, to cooperate with the nurses and doctors, and so on. The boy listened quietly and then asked, "Is it all right for me to feel a little homesick, too?"

THE WAYS PEOPLE REACTED TO POLIO and the sometimes extreme dislocation it caused in families was influenced by the social context of the times. In the United States during the 1940s and 1950s, a can-do spirit permeated the culture and helped form a value system for polio patients based on the power of individual will. Davis tells of one mother who, intending to encourage her own son, compared him to "a fellow down in Virginia" who had polio and was told he'd never get out of a wheelchair, but learned to walk with "just a little bit of a limp." The woman explained, "He just made up his mind he was going to do it himself." He tells of another mother, whose son recovered from polio with only minimal paralysis, who said: "It was his own wanting to and fighting against it that did it. He'd just talk about when he came home he was going to ride his bike, and, by gosh, he did." Such incidents as these, Davis wrote, add "to our culture's ample storehouse of myths, tales, and 'known instances' of man's triumphing over seemingly impossible circumstances to prove that it is he and he alone who fashions his fate. The improvement shown by these children became for the parents a miniature reenactment of the classic American success story." This goal-directedness was extreme enough to cause a systematic exaggeration of the difficulty of circumstances so that the individual could acquire "rather inexpensively," according to Davis, a feeling of accomplishment in the face of adversity.

The measured, steady quality of physical therapy gave a public demonstration of the individual's willpower to the patient, and to family and friends. In an essay based on a study of polio narratives, the historian Daniel J. Wilson contended that the patient and the physical therapist were bound "in the covenant of work," ensuring that the will to work remained strong even when results were meager. The treatment for paralytic polio was, according to Davis, "the quintessence of the Protestant ideology of achievement in America—namely, slow, patient, and regularly applied effort in pursuit of a long-range goal." "The gradient structuring of the physiotherapy regime tapped the deep and implicit faith of the families in the efficacy of 'will power' in overcoming adverse conditions," Davis wrote. The elaborate apparatus of physical therapy, with its gymnastic-type dumbbells, wall pulleys, and parallel bars, gave the impression that something was being done, whether the changes were significant or not. Parents in Davis's study, like the ones who counseled their children to cooperate with doctors and nurses, worried their children would be homesick in the hospital, not only because they didn't want them to be unhappy, but because they feared that if their children were miserable, they would be incapable of harnessing their willpower in behalf of recovery.

Writing about her friend Bea Wright, biographer Eleanor Chappell voiced the spirit expected of polio victims. When Wright got her diagnosis, according to Chappell, she knew that the "right way" to deal with it was to fight: "This was no sanctimonious weakling resolving to silently bear her burden, but a woman who refused to accept what had happened as a locked door." One woman I talked to who had polio in 1949 at age seven and learned to walk again, theorized recently that people who had polio in the postwar period took on the attitude of the war—"positive, uplifting, and fighting." And they had Franklin Roosevelt to look to as a symbol of strength and victory over polio so that "they didn't feel victimized by the disease." This woman said: "I never felt like a victim or ever felt that I wouldn't succeed in conquering polio. . . . I feel that if I just work hard enough and try with all my strength that I will be successful."

The symbol for triumph in the minds of many polio patients, their families, the public, and even some medical personnel was walking. Patients unable to breathe or sit up asked their physical therapists, "When am I going to walk?" Elizabeth Wheelwright, the physical therapist at the Northwest Respirator Center, told me when I telephoned her to talk again after meeting her at the picnic in Seattle, that in her work with polio patients she often became distressed over the emphasis placed on walking. These forty years later, her voice still hardened when she spoke of the patients who tried against terrible odds to walk and failed: "There was lots of damned guilt built up with the patient," she said.

Physical therapy was often successful in the first months of convalescence—a fact, Fred Davis said, that proved its later undoing.

Parents watching their children progress from bed to wheelchair and perhaps to ambulation began to see it as a cure attributed to physical therapy and to think that the hard work and therapy infused "life and motor force into damaged and destroyed muscles." Instead, wrote Davis, physical therapy, "and, for that matter, any other form of medical treatment of residual polio paralysis—is a method of rehabilitation and not a cure. The paralysis must be accepted as given and efforts made to work around it or to compensate for it; it cannot be done away with."

Often, it was only far into the treatment that the patient and the family began to see that the only realistic goal was compensation for the losses. Leonard Kriegel wrote that rehabilitation is "a thief's primer of compensation and deception: its purpose was to teach one how to steal a touch of the normal from an existence that would be striking in its abnormality." Rehabilitation meant integrating these new abilities—some of them radically different, depending on the extent of paralysis—into one's rewritten life story.

Some patients did exhibit incredible strength in trying to overcome the handicaps of polio, but for many, that was not enough. Roosevelt spent the first seven years of paralysis with walking as his principal interest and full-time occupation. He tried massage, salt-water baths, ultraviolet light, electric currents, parallel bars as supports, horseback riding, an electric tricycle, exercises in warm water and cold water, osteopathy, and every manner of muscle training. He exercised in the morning and practiced walking in the afternoon. Despite all that effort, time, and expense, he never managed more than a few tortured steps supported by braces, a cane, and the strong arm of someone else. In fact, he never even stood up, except for speeches, receptions, and military reviews.

In essays recounting his polio experience, Leonard Kriegel described his teenage efforts to learn to maneuver in the world with useless legs bound in full-length braces as he leaned on crutches. In a "cavernous room filled with barbells and Indian clubs and crutches and walkers" he built up his strength. In the hospital rehabilitation room he learned "to mount two large wooden steps made to the exact measure of a New York City bus's." He wrote: "I would swing on parallel bars from one side to the other, my arms learning how they would have to hurl me through the world." He did hundreds of push-ups daily to build up his arms, shoulders, and chest; he did dips on the monkey bars for hours at a time to create triceps strong enough to carry him "endlessly through the days and nights of [his] need."

NOT ALL PATIENTS WERE CAPABLE of demonstrating—or willing to demonstrate—their grit with physical feats, the way the teenaged Kriegel did. Dorothy Pallas was seven in 1939 when she came down with a severe case of polio that left her without a hope of walking. She wrote years later that sometime during the next seven years, spent in and out of hospitals, without knowing it, she made a decision.

> I could not put all my energy into getting well. I wanted too much to live and do things, whether or not I moved again. I knew some patients who learned to take a few struggling steps using braces and crutches and never got any further. I saw the tremendous energy that this required, and I wondered where so few steps could take them.
>
> Perhaps the thing that held me back from thinking such thoughts openly was fear of being called a quitter and a coward, the one who couldn't take it. I was accused of that as it was. I screamed during back-bending and hell-stretching, a disgrace to my braver companions, the ones with 'grit.' . . . At any rate, I know now that, rightly or wrongly, I divided my strength between treatments . . . and making do."

Pallas, and who knows how many others who struggled through physical therapy, felt a finger point at them, insisting they try harder, do more, be more. Brody explains this don't-let-it-beat-you expectation society has of the ill (and handicapped), and they have of themselves, by saying that illness is "a form of socially deviant behavior," so the rest of us approve of the sick person who "tries hard to get well" because that shows an effort to abandon "the deviance and return to the socially valued state." And so, polio patients grappled with the dilemma of dividing their time between getting better and living life. Some found, as my mother's friend Helen Willie told me she did, that trying to walk with braces took time and energy that she needed for her family life instead. And so she gave up her braces and conducted her life from her wheelchair.

The more polio stories I heard, the more I saw this desire to believe that individual will can overpower any hardship as a hollow aim. The public view of polio seemed to be a collective refutation of what polio really did to people and their lives. The by-gosh-he-did-it outlook, the need to believe that human will can overcome *anything*, diminished the profound experiences of many patients.

No one worked harder than the NFIP to foster the idea that polio could be beaten. In one of its "Strange Facts about Polio," a political-cartoon-like feature that ran in newspapers, for example, the NFIP explained frog breathing as a technique that allowed polio victims to leave their iron lungs, sometimes for hours. True enough, but the accompanying drawing showed an empty iron lung and a pretty, smiling woman—presumably the patient—sitting nearby sipping from a coffee mug. The implication was that iron-lung patients, being as well and healthy as that woman with her dark pageboy, popped in and out of their iron lungs at will, and sat around sipping hot drinks. The reality was far different for most respiratory patients, who usually had other paralysis to go along with their limited breathing power. And frog breathing, as my mother's case shows, was not a given, but a hard-won, difficult skill.

In Daniel Wilson's examination of more than fifty published "polio narratives," accounts of polio victims, he found that almost all of them were structured as tales of triumph over adversity. The patients who succumbed to the disease, through death or failure to progress in rehabilitation or failure to adjust to limited abilities, were either not mentioned at all or only in passing. My family's story is one of those dismissed by the insistence to see triumph. Those of us in my family who were untouched physically and my mother, who was,

could not overcome the obstacles polio presented us. My family's polio story is a tale without heroes and without victory.

BELIEVING, OR PRETENDING, that each ounce of effort or will
or desire had a payback didn't account for the extreme incapacities
polio could deliver. Wilson noted that "the failure to beat polio physically often produced depression and despair. . . . Not surprisingly,
those most severely disabled, and especially those needing breathing
assistance, experienced the deepest dejection." What was a severely
paralyzed patient like my mother to think of herself in a milieu that
demanded the triumph of will over adversity?

"My breathing was labored," wrote Regina Woods of her first
days with the disease that left her a respiratory quadriplegic. "I could
move nothing, and I had no idea what was happening to me. I was
surrounded by strangers who kept telling me to 'try,' a word that I
came to hate. I didn't understand, because nothing moved and I
didn't know how to *try* to breathe. I had always just done it."

Without doubt, the plight of respiratory patients, like Woods
and my mother, were the most difficult for both the public and the
individual to deal with. In my effort to understand the emotional
repercussions of polio, particularly as they might apply to my mother,
I searched out studies of respiratory patients. One, done in 1952 on
eighteen respirator patients at the Mary MacArthur Respirator Unit
of the Children's Hospital in Boston, found that despite differences in
personality structure before the onset of polio, reactions to the illness, at least for those with breathing problems, followed a common
pattern.

Patients went through three overlapping, distinguishable stages
as they learned to assimilate and adjust to the catastrophic effects of
their illness. The researchers observed that the patients first regressed to
infantile behaviors and thoughts, a reaction fostered by the regression
in physical dependence to a babyish state in which all or most bodily
needs had to be met by someone else. Reading this, I was reminded of
the confusion Arnold Beisser faced with the contrast between the man
he was and the infant dependency he had returned to. "Nurses and

attendants often talked to me as if I were a baby," he wrote. "If I be-came soiled . . . they were likely to say, 'Naughty, naughty,' or 'You've been a bad boy.' "

In this stage, which my mother experienced while she was hospitalized in Phoenix, the patient showed increased narcissism, had little energy to turn outward toward others, and used what psychiatrists call "infantile mechanisms of adaption," such as denial and primitive fantasies. Many patients, even those unable to breathe or move, spoke of being on their feet again, of riding a bicycle again. They had dreams in which they were perfectly well and walking normally.

In the second stage, patients experienced one or several peri-ods of depression of varying intensity, in the process of facing their situation. In this stage patients became irritable and demanding, and felt disliked and unwanted. With no radical transformation in her physical condition forthcoming, my mother floundered in Seattle, sinking into depression. "I worried about her," was the first comment Fred Plum made when I telephoned him to ask if he remembered caring for her in Seattle. "She cried a good deal of the time." Marcelle Dunning said she thought my mother's severe physical handicaps robbed her of the energy and emotional strength to imagine a future for herself. It was, Dunning said, as if her imagination were frozen.

This was an understandably difficult period for the patient, the family, and the staff. Patients took issue with trivial matters, such as how a sheet was laid on the bed or how many minutes of physio-therapy were given. Patients viewed such matters as indicators of how others valued them. They became bossy, uncooperative, and hostile in their efforts to ward off depression. During the struggle of this second stage, according to the researchers, "the attitudes of families and of the staff members, as family surrogates, were especially impor-tant . . . since the patient[s] tended to interpret illness as punishment . . . and were sensitive to any behavior on the part of others which might be considered rejection."

I was grateful that by the time I read this study and learned how important the staff was to the well-being of the patient, I had met some of my mother's Seattle caregivers. I had assumed that the people who volunteered to work with polio patients, and especially with the hard cases in respirator centers, must have had a measure of compassion and devotion to their profession that kept them from choosing more peaceful duty. They had to work extraordinarily hard, and sometimes even the good ones could fall short. There were good-natured and attractive nurses who were nonetheless dreaded by patients because they couldn't give a sponge bath without soaking the bed linens. And the worst of the caregivers were a disaster. Patients joked about the dim-witted helpers, like the one who threw a blanket over the iron lung when the patient inside complained of cold. They joked, but they also must have been furious.

Careful attention given by the good caregivers could help patients overcome depression and feelings of rejection. A patient at the Northwest Respirator Center reported in "The Vital Capacitor" about an outing several patients enjoyed to the nurses' building for a variety show, with music, dancing, and magic. But the patients appreciated almost as much the fact that after the show the student nurses accompanied the patients back to the center and put them to bed for the night. Each patient had three or four attendants that night devoted to providing him or her the most assiduous service. Each patient was lavishly washed, given his nightly range-of-motion exercises, and left to "pleasant memories of the occasion," the report said. The attention was "a kindness that [the patients would] not soon forget."

IN THE FRAGILE EMOTIONAL and physical state of respiratory patients especially, caregivers boosted or depleted faltering self-esteem. Simply keeping a quadriplegic's discomfort within tolerable limits can be a tedious and time-consuming job. As Gene Roehling wrote, "My whole comfort depends on just how much effort [the nurses] want to put forth. . . . Pain is something you don't get used to, so I keep trying for the relief from it." Arnold Beisser wrote of the "blind rage" he felt when he asked a nurse for a blanket to cover his paralyzed, shivering body. The nurse touched his leg and said, "Oh, it's all right, you're not cold." With such callous helpers, Beisser felt "like an undeserving outsider—regarded at best with curiosity, but usually with disinterest or disdain."

The best of the caregivers gave willingly with interest and compassion and seemed to be nurtured by their relationships with people who needed them, wrote Arnold Beisser, and with them he felt "restored to the human community." The best of them performed duties that ranged from life-saving—rushing to a bedside and pumping a failed iron lung, for example—to simple acts that helped patients find dignity and self-respect, even for the moment. One physician, for example, interrupted his schedule to give Beisser a much-needed shave. With or without good care, however, respiratory patients passed into depression, which surely made even the best of caregivers falter in their dedication.

The third stage was the process of adaptation. This was, of course, ongoing and lengthy, continuing long after a patient's discharge from the hospital. It was during this stage that greater individual differences showed up, when whatever psychological difficulties that had existed in the person when he or she became ill came into play.

In this vague, sometimes vast, area between depression and acceptance, some patients found what Wilson calls "grace." In the polio narratives he studied, he found the themes of recovery and redemption, which he likened to the Puritan covenants of work and grace. Work was the patient's physical therapy, but at "some point in every case, constraints appeared," he wrote. "The extent of the destruction became apparent; progress in recovery slowed or came to a halt." Just as the Puritans believed they could not earn salvation through their good works alone, paralyzed polio patients found they needed something else—and that, Wilson says, was the covenant of grace, the achievement of "some level of understanding, some sense of acceptance and resignation."

For most who achieved grace—and not all did—the process was "a protracted and difficult struggle against physical limitations and psychological scars," wrote Wilson. "Physical therapists and doctors did all they could to restore the body, but the person had to look to inner resources to restore the mind and spirit." Only through this phenomenon of grace, whether its roots were sacred or secular, could patients revise the stories of their lives.

Perhaps the biggest obstacle to acceptance was the much-touted expectation that anyone could, through hard work, be restored to the previous undamaged self. Even the news of Sister Kenny's miracles and the NFIP's ballyhooed successes must have undermined those struggling to accept the unchangeable. Victims and their families spent months, even years, in doubt about what long-term effects polio might have. That was, in part, a result of the individual ways in which the disease worked and the limits of what medical science could tell them. But it was also because caregivers were reluctant, sometimes for good reason, to bear bad news.

DURING THE EARLY STAGES OF POLIO, medical people could not predict outcomes with any certainty. But as the weeks and months went on, extensive examination of muscles revealed much about the patient's prognosis. By the end of six weeks to three months, muscles were showing rapid return of strength, had moderate or little strength, or were still paralyzed. By then, the spinal motor cells either had or had not recovered their function. Destroyed nerve cells cannot be reproduced, so patients did well or poorly in proportion to the number of motor cells the disease spared.

By observing patients' progress following the acute phase of the disease, physicians and physiotherapists could make accurate predictions about the degree to which the patient's muscle capacity was likely to return. Nonetheless, doctors were loath to reveal their predictions to patients, unless, of course, complete recovery was expected. Davis found that the greater the probable handicap, the greater the reluctance to break the news. In his study, the probable progress of a handicapped child was "rarely" brought to the attention of the family before discharge. Instead, he found, "it was at best remotely alluded to or vaguely implied by treatment personnel, but never openly discussed." Many hospitals deliberately tried to avoid challenging or openly discouraging the parents' hopes and expectations for a perfect or near-perfect recovery. They preferred to let the family find out for themselves, believing they would eventually accept the handicap and somehow make the best of it. Medical personnel who were intentionally vague thought that with their silence and evasion they were sparing the stricken the shock of hearing bad news. They thought that in time the news would slowly, and less painfully, dawn on the crippled person and his or her family.

When I began my research and first encountered this issue of what doctors knew when and what they chose to tell patients, my views were too simple to cover the intricacies involved. I kept wanting doctors and patients to "face reality." I kept thinking that doctors should have told patients all they knew about their conditions as soon as possible, and that patients should have quickly begun living their lives reshaped by the truth of whatever new limitations faced them. I wanted clarity and found instead complexity.

I found that even when physicians wanted to say what could be expected of the patient, often they either failed to explain clearly or the families and patients failed to understand. One doctor in Davis's study noted, several weeks before a nine-year-old girl's discharge: "Maximum improvement has been reached, . . . [and] any further progress will be minimal. Her leg will remain flail." But almost three months later when the researchers interviewed the girl's mother, she was still expecting the doctors to, at any time, take away the girl's long brace and give her a short one instead. A year later the mother was still talking about the possibility of complete recovery, although her daughter was still wearing the long brace and using crutches, and had made no significant progress since her hospital discharge.

A period of about fifteen months after the onset of polio was generally viewed by caregivers as the time in which compensatory skills, depending on the patient's condition, could be developed. Doctors also saw that time period as a reasonable one in which the family could adjust to or accept whatever permanent handicap might remain, and thus most of the families in Davis's study were told (without much explanation) that "no further recovery could be expected after a period of 12 to 18 months from onset of the disease," usually meaning about six to twelve months after discharge from the hospital. Families, Davis found, often misinterpreted this to mean that if improvement hadn't yet taken place, it still might, "all of a sudden and in one or two great bursts, 'before the time [ran] out.' " For some, the fact that they had progressed at all was interpreted to mean that they would continue indefinitely to improve until, according to Davis, "some magical moment in the future when [they] would no longer be handicapped, incapacitated, or in any way different from [their] fellows." FDR, many years after becoming paralyzed, continued to speak of full recovery coming in two more years. One of his biographers, Hugh Gregory Gallagher, who also had polio, wrote: "Intellectually, he knew this was untrue. Emotionally, however, he found it hard to admit; politically . . . it served him to believe it to be true."

I began to see that the issue of telling patients what to expect was rife with pain and difficulty. That was partly so because, as Davis wrote, to be crippled is not merely a physical attribute of the person, but "in our culture it is also an important social fact about the person, carrying with it numerous social disadvantages." Because of the complex implications of what crippling meant to one's life story, mistakes were made by doctors and other medical personnel in delivering or not delivering the news and on the part of patients and their families in hearing the news. Children often did not or could not understand the physical or social implications of their conditions. One seven-year-old boy in Davis's study, two months out of the hospital with his legs in heavy braces, asked the Little League coach if he could be on the team. Not knowing what to say, the coach told the boy the positions were filled and he should ask again next year. The boy went home and joyfully told his mother: "I'll be playing with the Little Leaguers next year."

For physicians, the ones charged with telling patients and their families the prognosis, there seemed no good way to convey the permanence of crippling. One day Lou Sternburg, fully paralyzed, rocking on a bed, confronted his physician by asking, "When am I going to walk out of here?" The doctor looked embarrassed, his face flushed, and he let the rest of the group making rounds go on to another patient before replying: "We, er . . . we don't believe you'll ever walk again, Lou. And I may as well tell you that I don't think you'll ever breathe again without mechanical assistance." Lou asked him to repeat the statement. The doctor did, and then Lou screamed, as loudly as a respirator patient can, and said: "You sonofabitch, you're lying! . . . One of these days, I'm going to walk into your office and smack you right in the teeth!" "I hope you do," the doctor said. "I'm sorry, Lou."

When the truth was devastating, no wonder physicians avoided saying the words and patients refused to accept them. What my early impatience for directness and clarity from physicians failed to account for was that there is a limit to how much loss a human mind and heart can embrace at once. Again and again I was moved and humbled by hearing from polio survivors who were grateful that no one had made them face their changed conditions before they were ready. One woman told me that her ignorance of the truth in the early months of polio saved her sanity.

As I continued to read about and talk to polio survivors and their families, I slowly began to see how valuable, even vital, denial was as a survival technique. Denial is a safe place to rest while waiting for grace. Leonard Kriegel wrote of his early dependence on fantasy:

> I suppose we might have been told that our fall from grace was permanent. But I am still grateful that no one . . . told me that my chances of regaining the use of my legs were nonexistent. Like every other boy on the ward, I organized my needs around whatever illusions were available. And the illusion I needed above any other was that one morning I would simply wake up and rediscover the 'normal' boy of memory, once again playing baseball in French Charley's Field in Bronx Park. . . . At the age of eleven, I needed to weather reality, not face it. And to this very day I silently thank those who were concerned enough about me, or indifferent enough to my fate, not to tell me what they knew.

Even after the explosive scene with his doctor, Sternburg kept his blinders on. Someone took him for an outing to the golf course he had played before becoming ill. Being there didn't take him down, because he still thought that one day he'd play golf again, although by then he had conceded it might be from a wheelchair. Like most other severely disabled polio patients, Sternburg accepted his physical devastation only in stages, guided by some inner psychological regulator that allowed in only as much as he could endure. As he digested each bite of the larger truth, his regulator allowed in another measured amount, until one day he knew he would not only never play golf again, but would never again breathe unaided, never move a muscle below his neck.

H. C. A. Lassen, the chief physician in the department of communicable diseases at Blegdam Hospital in Copenhagen in the early 1950s wrote of the importance of psychological support for respirator patients after the acute stage when "the fully conscious patient faces a period of unpredictable length in the respirator. Although these patients usually have astonishingly good morale and fighting spirit, everything humanely possible should be done to keep it up. Untimely prognostications should be avoided, as it is practically never too late for the patient to realize he is a respirator patient for life."

Those words—"never too late for the patient to realize he is a respirator patient for life"—ran over and over in my mind, a wash of common sense and humanity, and I wondered whether my mother had been unable to deny her condition sufficiently. Did she contemplate, while still in the respirator center, the full range of what "for life" could mean? Is that what held her in depression? Had her internal regulator failed her and allowed in a larger portion than she could handle?

Her emotional frailty and the truth of that never-too-late philosophy was demonstrated poignantly for me in a story I read in a 1951 issue of the *Saturday Evening Post* by Gene Roehling. Still in an iron lung after two years, he was able only to squeeze his buttocks together, shrug his shoulders slightly, and move a finger of his left hand. He was quoted as saying:

> Obviously I don't like living in this thing and having
> my insides connected up permanently to a battery of
> bottles and tubes, and there have been black times

when I think I might have just quietly turned the darned thing off if I had been able. But I live one day now, and when that's over I go to work on the next one, and certainly I don't burn my heart with thoughts about how it all might have been. I usually don't think about the future at all, and if I have to, I consider it in a detached sort of way, and it seems to me that the future is of necessity a series of steps.

The first step for him, he determined, was to learn to breathe on his own. "Time has lost much of its significance, and if it sometimes seems that I am spending too much time on the bottom step, I don't get discouraged. . . . I came to this situation with what is probably the ideal mental equipment; I think neither very much nor very deeply."

Hearing the detachment in those lines, I knew that to force someone in his situation to consider his long-range prospects would have been unspeakably cruel. I could not go back to my rigid line of thinking that held "facing reality" above all else. "Weathering reality," Kriegel's term and tactic, while one tried to compose a new life narrative, fit the situation for many polio survivors far better.

Like the patients, family members were also affected emotionally and psychologically. Being singled out in the random way the disease traveled threatened a family's view of itself and required the family to abandon the protective notion that calamity befalls others, not us. Like the patients, families needed to protect themselves from too large a dose of misery with a kind of collective mechanism akin to the individual's internal regulator. They needed time to absorb the sometimes profound implications of their loved one's incapacity. They, too, had suffered severe ruptures in the stories of their lives and needed time to rewrite the narratives to accommodate the new facts—a son in a wheelchair, perhaps, or a wife on a rocking bed. I found that my family's inability or unwillingness to talk about the crippling of my mother—to her, to others, among themselves—was far from unusual. Jack Clements's wife, Bette, came down with a severe case of polio in September 1955, when she was twenty-one and he twenty-three. Through her nearly two years of hospitalization, he visited her daily; but he never discussed her prognosis with her, and she never asked about it. "It's a cliché," Clements wrote to me, "but we did take everything one day at a time." Even when she returned home, still fully paralyzed, they kept her clothes and shoes and other personal items around the house for when she got well. "We both knew this was a fantasy," he wrote, "but 'pretended' this would happen 'some day,' although we never actually discussed it." The couple were coping as best they could with the radically altered life polio had foisted upon them. If knowing her shoes still waited in her closet brought even a tiny measure of comfort to Bette, then certainly that's where her shoes should have been.

POLIO SURVIVORS WRESTLED not only with considerable internal turmoil in trying to integrate the life changes paralysis demanded, but also with the pressures of external expectations. If time and hard work failed to restore the polio patient, then society expected patients to bear their trials silently. A social taboo that forbade the disabled from expressing bitterness, pain, disappointment, anger, and anguish, except superficially, was well in place by the 1940s and guided the polio patient. In one of the stories for popular magazines that Ken Purdy wrote about his son Geoff's illness, he told of a girl Geoff met during his stay at Warm Springs who could move nothing but her fingers. Although Geoff visited with her nightly, she never once mentioned her disability, something Purdy related with apparent approval. It's approval, I'd say, for her behavior as a "good handicapped person." The concept, as outlined by the physician Howard Brody and employed in Daniel Wilson's study, means that the disabled person should not dwell on the disability or indulge in self-pity or any attitude that suggests resignation to life with a handicap. Instead, the person's life should be "devoted to an enthusiastic and diligent struggle against [the] handicapping condition," and the person should seek "every opportunity for normal function, achievement, and happiness." The disabled person should try as hard as possible to create a life and career, ideally attaining some position one would not expect a paralyzed person to be able to occupy.

Although the disabled people in the published polio narratives Wilson studied had adhered to the social mores of good handicapped people, his examination of letters polio patients had written to President Roosevelt, contained in the FDR library at Hyde Park, suggested that depression and anger were widespread. Roosevelt himself suffered depression that he kept hidden even from those closest to him.

One of my correspondents, Betty Hurwich Zoss, told me of a friend, Harriet, who had been completely paralyzed by polio and had gone home to try to live her life and raise her children despite her condition. Acquaintances said of Harriet, "She never ever said a word of complaint or felt sorry for herself." "Sorry!" Zoss told me, "She was furious, bless her, and told me so. Those who thought they were praising her just didn't know her." But the attitude others saw in Harriet, because they wanted to, was of the good handicapped person who didn't cause embarrassment or discomfort in the able-bodied by expressing difficult emotions.

Writing in the fifties of his son's experience with polio in both *McCall's* and *Reader's Digest* magazines, Ken Purdy showed repeatedly that his son took naturally to the good handicapped role. Purdy quoted his son as saying when he first saw his parents after his isolation period: "I don't feel so bad. I've felt worse than this. . . . Of course, my legs are dead, but the rest of me is alive." Writing to a friend, Purdy said of his son's morale: "[It] approaches the incredible, and he has yet to be heard to say that it's too bad this happened to him or anything like that. The farthest he's gone is to say that he had a bad summer this year. . . . He has put up quite an astonishing show for a 12-year-old."

That word *show* was a telling choice, indicating that even the proud father must have known that beneath the good cheer, surely, was pain. I can't help but think that Geoff's chin-up attitude, brave and heartening as it was, was just the beginning. Although the rest of him was alive, surely those dead legs would eventually give him reason to grieve.

A counterpoint view came to me through James Warwick, whose brother, Bill, lived for more than twenty years able to move nothing more than the fingers on one hand slightly and to wag a foot.

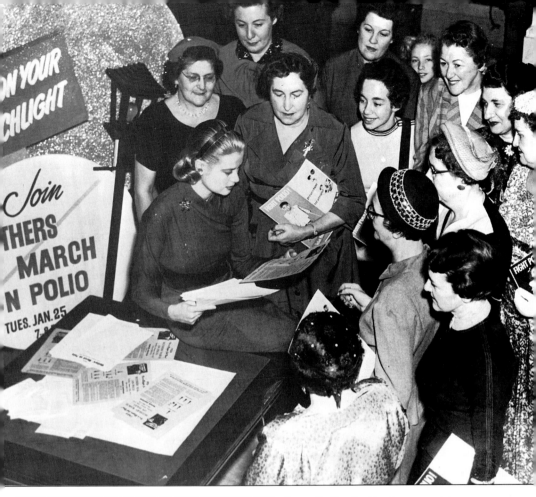

Grace Kelly distributing materials to Mothers March on Polio leaders in Philadelphia, December 1954
(*March of Dimes Birth Defects Foundation*)

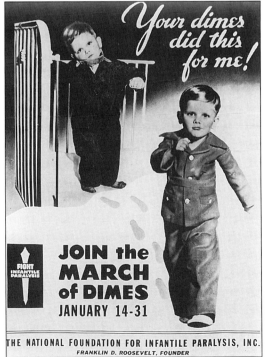

Donald Anderson, first March of Dimes poster child, 1946
(*March of Dimes Birth Defects Foundation*)

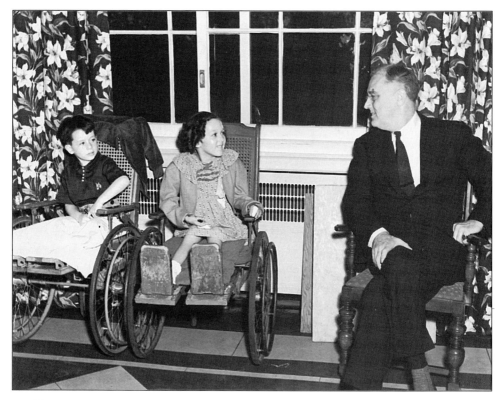

Franklin D. Roosevelt and patients at Georgia Warm Springs (*March of Dimes Birth Defects Foundation*)

Patients at Georgia Warm Springs exercising under the supervision of physical therapists (*March of Dimes Birth Defects Foundation*)

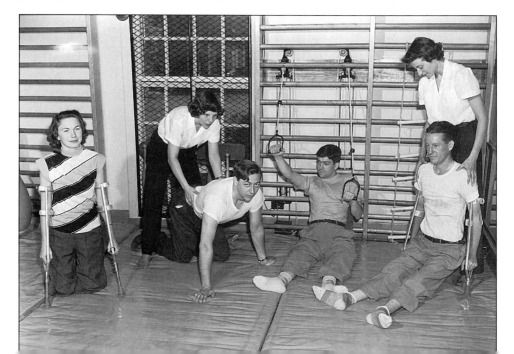

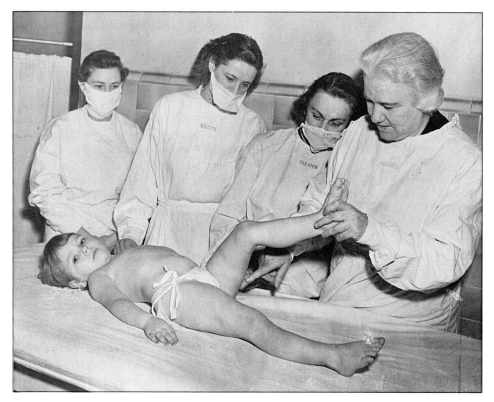

Elizabeth Kenny demonstrating her techniques at the Sister Kenny Institute in Minneapolis, mid–1940s (*Minnesota Historical Society*)

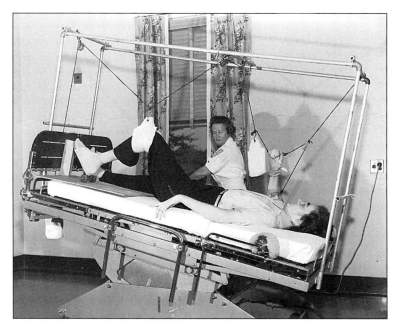

Polio patient exercising on a rocking bed, D.T. Watson School in Pennsylvania (*March of Dimes Birth Defects Foundation*)

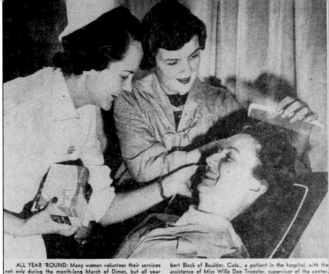

ALL YEAR 'ROUND: Many women volunteer their services not only during the month-long March of Dimes, but all year long. Some of them work in the Northwest Respirator Center in Harborview County Hospital. Mrs. F. W. Ecker, center, chairman of the center's volunteers, gave a permanent to Mrs. Delbert Black of Boulder, Colo., a patient in the hospital, with the assistance of Miss Willa Dee Troester, supervisor of the center. Mrs. Black, mother of two children, spent three months in an iron lung and now is aided by a portable Monaghan respirator. —Times staff photo by Larry Dion

Newspaper clipping of Virginia Black with nurse Willa Dee Troester and volunteer Mrs. F. W. Ecker at the Northwest Respirator Center, Seattle, January 30, 1955 (*Seattle Times*)

Polio Patient to Rejoin Children

Last September, Mrs. Delbert Black, a 29-year-old mother, lost the companionship of her two children and acquired that of a machine.

Yesterday, Mrs. Black left Seattle to fly back to her children. But the machine went along. She never may be able to live without it.

Mrs. Black has not seen the children since she was struck down by paralytic poliomyelitis September 21 in Phoenix.

Paralyzed from the neck down, Mrs. Black was placed in an iron lung and flown to the Northwest Respirator Center in Harborview County Hospital.

Her husband, a loan-company employee, has visited her several times in the hospital here. But the children, Kenneth, 7, and Kathy, 5, could not come.

"We were just preparing to move from Phoenix back to Boulder, Colo., where I was born and raised, when polio struck," said Mrs. Black.

"Now, at last, I can go home again. I can see my children again."

Mrs. Black was brought here because the respirator center nearest her, in Los Angeles, was full. She was flown to Denver yesterday in a specially equipped Military Air Transport Service plane.

Her constant companion henceforth will be an electrically operated portable respirator. The respirator can be operated by hand in case of a power failure.

After a few days in Denver General Hospital, Mrs. Black will go home to Boulder to begin an unfamiliar life in a familiar setting.

GOING HOME: Mrs. Delbert Black of Boulder, Colo., paralyzed from the neck down by poliomyelitis, smiled as she prepared to leave the Northwest Respirator Center in Harborview County Hospital yesterday. Mrs. Cecil Bell, nurse, adjusted controls on Mrs. Black's portable respirator.

Kin of Dreiser Dies

NEW YORK, June 11. — (N. Y. News)—Mrs. Mai V. Dreiser, 76, sister-in-law of the Theodore Dreiser, late novelist, died today

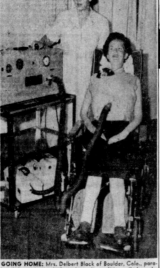

Del and Virginia at the Northwest Respirator Center, Seattle, c. 1955 (*Author collection*)

Newspaper clipping of Virginia preparing to leave the Northwest Respirator Center, June 12, 1955 (*Seattle Times*)

Kathy and Kenny in front of Maurine and Hayes Royce's house, Boulder, April 1955 (*Author collection*)

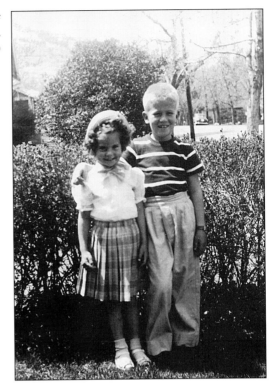

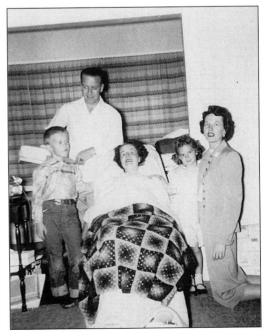

Newspaper clipping showing Virginia's reunion with Kenny and Kathy in Denver, June 13, 1955 (*Denver Post*)

Kenny, Del, Kathy, and Katherine Donald gathered around Virginia in her wheelchair, in the house on Tenth Street, c. 1956 (*Author collection*)

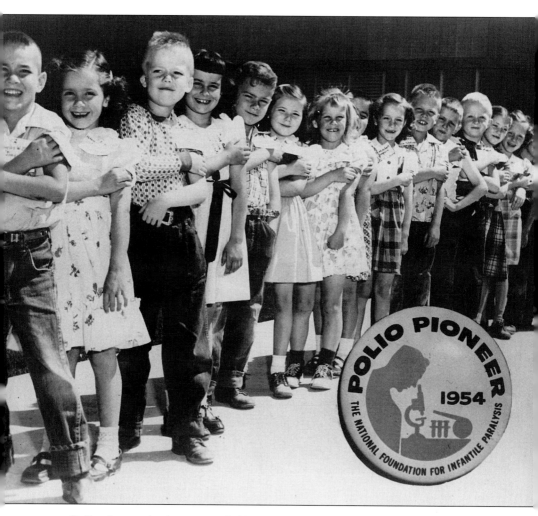

Polio pioneers in the vaccine field trials, 1954 (*March of Dimes Birth Defects Foundation*)

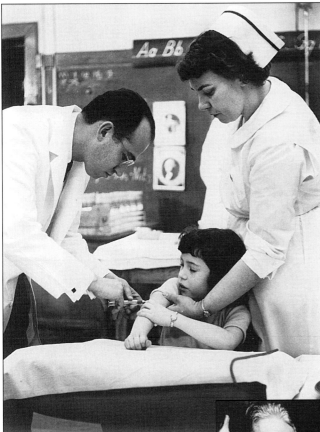

Jonas Salk administering the Salk polio vaccine at Colfax School, Pittsburgh, 1954 (*March of Dimes Birth Defects Foundation*)

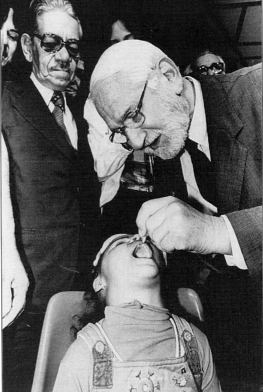

Albert Sabin administering his oral polio vaccine (*WHO/Pasteur Merieux*)

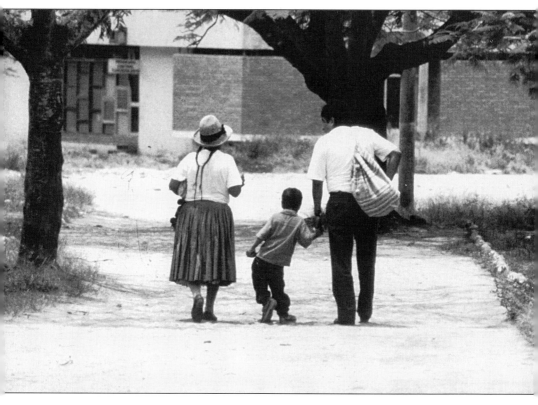

Luis Fermin Tenorio, the last polio case in the Western Hemisphere (*WHO/PAHO/A. Waak*)

James told me he never heard Bill "bemoan his fate, he never was ill humored, indeed, he had a marvelous sense of understated humor. He would kid about having the bottom of his shoes, as well as the top, shined." He wrote to friends on cards propped on his chest, using a pen that had been placed in his mouth, and often concluded by saying his jaw was getting tired. He spent a lifetime speaking to public groups, having learned to talk all over again in a voice his brother described as "strange but mesmerizing." In his speeches he challenged his audiences to use their mobility, saying, for example: "Well, all of you pedestrians, where have you walked lately?" or "How many of you can raise your right arm? Now your left? OK, having shown me that, how many of you have hugged your kids today?" He used the line long before it became a bumper-sticker slogan. But once during a visit when his brother complained about something, Bill replied, "Do you want to swap? You give me your worst day, and I'll give you my best—what do you say?" Bill's refusal to dismiss, discount, or ignore his condition apparently only enhanced the affection and regard of others. James concluded one letter to me about his brother, who died in 1978, with: "I miss him very much," and the next letter: "But enough, the memories are too painful."

Society also had expectations of families—again, expectations at odds with reality. Families were to play their roles, Davis observed in his study, with a "blend of sorrow, courage, altruism, and solidarity that American mores define as appropriate in such situations." Families told researchers that they had found greater solidarity and amity in their family life now that they had a sick child. One mother, for example, said of her crippled boy, "With this happening, I guess we just wouldn't think of arguing or saying anything to each other, because we feel like nothing is important except Marvin." But in a later interview she complained that her husband didn't earn enough money to support the family well, that close relatives neglected and avoided the family, and that the younger child was selfish and demanding during the ill child's absence. Even in families who were genuinely drawn closer by polio, the researchers observed, "strains and tensions soon became evident in . . . most of the families."

Family members coped with guilt, anxiety, shame, embarrassment, depression, resentment, rejection, alienation, self-blame, and bitterness. In one recent study, researchers found that families with a chronically ill child felt strained under their limited mobility and financial burdens, which heightened feelings of guilt and resentment in the parents and constricted the relationships between the healthy children and the ill one. Families with an ill or handicapped member, according to Brody, "are at a high risk for a feeling of meaninglessness, a feeling of being cut off from their community and their culture." Often families, like the patients, floundered in their efforts to adapt to new roles and changed life stories.

WHEN I LOOKED into the social and psychological experience of polio, I encountered duality and contradiction, but I also found a consistency: the only way out of the maze of social expectations and personal suffering for both family members and the polio survivor lay in hope. I came to see that the diverse ways people coped with what polio left them were individual efforts to grasp hope, whether in stoicism, cheerfulness, fantasy, religious faith, or physical feats. Denial, too, seemed to be an effort to cling to hope. Perhaps the role of that internal regulator, which allowed in only measured doses of manageable psychological pain, was to preserve hope.

Patients paralyzed by polio needed not only the will to make the most of their remaining muscle strength, but a belief that all would yet be well, that the future might yet fulfill desire. The hope they needed was not based on the facile notion of the power of positive thinking, but on the fundamentally human ability to look forward with desire to a future that is not yet visible, but is possible. For those who faced a life changed by physical limitations, hope could rest not on expecting a cure but on finding usefulness, physical and emotional, and then value in the life one has.

I don't know whether my mother could do that. I don't know whether she had the means—time, education, faith, whatever it took—to evolve to a place where she could find a measure of peace in the passive, dependent life polio left her. Her losses were staggering. She could do nothing she had done in the past, none of the acts that defined her, except talk, think, and listen. She was forced in the starkest way to find meaning for her life in being, not doing.

Had I the power to know what her thoughts and feelings were as she prepared to leave Seattle and go home to what her life had become, perhaps I would find that she had transformed her condition into something meaningful. Perhaps not. I can only hope that she had enough wishing power left to anticipate with some pleasure the life awaiting her in Colorado.

CHAPTER SEVEN

Forgetting and Remembering

Two young school-age children, a boy and a girl, ran around and around in the bright lights of an air force landing base calling out, "Hi, Mommy! Hi, Mommy!" as a C-47 troop carrier landed. The rear loading door of the airplane, designed to carry nearly thirty soldiers, opened to the summer night air and released its single passenger and her attendants. In a deeply reclined wheelchair, a battery for the portable respirator in tow, the woman was pushed across the tarmac to her family: grandparents, parents, an aunt and a cousin, and her two gleeful children. Her husband was not present, but emergency medical crews, a fire engine, and a crowd of hospital and air force personnel gathered to aid and watch, curious about this unusual flight. At the woman's request, her cousin had selected, bought, and wrapped gifts, happy-to-see-you-again presents for the two children she'd been separated from for over a year.

THE WOMAN, OF COURSE, IS MY MOTHER; the children, Kenny and me; the reunion, ours in 1955. We've come to the part of my family's story in which Mother's and my paths merge again, and yet I feel as distant from that coming together as if I were hearing the reunion story of some other five-year-old dimpled daughter and her mother. I couldn't write the scene in first person because I don't remember it. Not a happy skip nor nervous, expectant first sighting of the cargo door swinging open and not the smile I hope was on my mother's face. Nothing of that night remains for me. But how can it be that after a year away from her, I can't remember my first sight of her face? Here in our family narrative when Mother came back to us for what would be only a short time, here where I wanted and expected to find intimacy, I found distance.

All along in my effort to put together this narrative, to discover what polio did to Mother and, ultimately, to our family, I sought help from others to fill in the myriad essential facts I didn't or couldn't know because I wasn't there to see for myself or was too young to understand what I saw. But at this point in the chronology, with Mother back in Colorado, in a house I shared with her, among people I knew then and know now, my expectations were different. I thought I could enter the story and tell of her with my own memories. I thought I could tell of *us*. But I was wrong. I was there, but not there. There, but not significant. There, but too confused for events to register in my memory. There, but not really in Mother's story at all.

I've probed for memories, breaking the silence that long surrounded that time and my mother, sometimes stirring emotions that had been buried for decades. I asked, presuming an intimacy with my family that didn't exist. I asked, and in doing so, I gathered anecdotes, scraps of factual information, a few points of conjecture to add to my own. From them I tried to build a framework around this time and its events. I think of it as building a picket fence to order the bits and pieces and to contain, or at least surround, the confusion and suffering of my family during those months. I pound in the pickets, but they are too few and the gaps too many, and I see that it's a sorry fence.

When I sat down to write of this time, I thought of it as the period when Mother was "home again," and that was the working title I assigned this chapter. But, once again, I was wrong. I was wrong to think of Mother's return as a homecoming, in the sense of a return to what is remembered, loved, comfortable. For Mother, it was far less a going back to her former life than an entry into the strange and unknown. Her surroundings were familiar, the neighborhood where she grew up, but in almost every other way she faced the unfamiliar. The house that waited for her in Boulder was a rented one, the home of a friend and neighbor where Mother had visited but never expected to live. It wasn't Mother's home with her dishes arranged in the cupboards and her shoes in the closet where she had left them. She, most of all, was changed, but her parents and children were different, too, transformed as she was by time, by her illness and absence.

Another part of the homecoming misconception I had to raze was thinking of this as a joyful time. The joy didn't even survive the night of Mother's arrival. The medical personnel who waited for her at Lowry Air Force Base came with the intention of taking her to Colorado General Hospital in Denver to put her into an iron lung. She hadn't known that would happen. The doctors wanted to be sure she adjusted to the thin air of Colorado's mile-high altitude after spending the last eight months at sea level. So that night, Maurine, Hayes, Kenny, and I went back to Boulder without her, and Mother returned to the confining tank she had fought so hard to be free of.

The next day, a Sunday, the four of us drove the thirty miles back to Denver to visit Mother at the hospital. And that I do remember. It was the only time I saw her in an iron lung. When I first began to talk to my father about our family, I told him I remembered seeing Mother in a tank respirator, and he said, kindly enough, but firmly, that I had not. Yet, in my mind's eye, I could see her in a room with others in iron lungs. Her head, lying on the tray of her tank, was almost eye-level with me, and I *remember* seeing her from a distance, across a room. I wanted to be close to her, to touch her, but the memory freezes there, like a photograph. I remember nothing that anyone said, but I can still see her head there, and her smile. She *was* smiling, but not at me. The smile pointed up, towards somewhere else. I thought she looked sick, but I wasn't afraid.

Only after talking to others and, over time, piecing together dates and sequences did I realize my memory was real. I even have proof: A newspaper reporter and photographer also visited Mother the day after her return to Colorado, and soon after, a story and photograph appeared in the *Denver Post*. Aunt Lourie clipped the story and put it in her diary, and at rare and unpredictable moments throughout grade school, I went next door to her house and asked to see it. She would take her 1955 diary from the drawer next to her reading chair and invite me to sit on her lap. As I leaned into her soft body, she'd hold the fragile, yellowed clipping, and I'd stare at the photograph. Yes, I'd had a mother, it reassured me. The photograph shows seven-year-old Kenny with a bristly crewcut and his shirt buttoned to the neck and five-year-old me with a bow in my hair, both of us smiling tentatively. Looking pleased but shy, we stand close to each other next to Mother in the iron lung. Kenny has one arm reaching around me, toward Mother's face. Now, when I look at the photograph, I see how well it captured our family as we were during the months that followed: Mother and her two children huddled close, not touching, waiting for our life to resume, and my father is absent. I also see that it is separate from the memory I hold of Mother in the iron lung. In the photo our faces are close; in my memory I am distant from her, watching her, unable to reach her.

I don't remember the newspaper reporter or photographer and have only a faded memory of Mother in the iron tank, but what I recall clearly about that Sunday in Denver was being outside the hospital, waiting.

For the rest of the afternoon, until the sun began to fade and the lights in the hospital came on, Kenny and I played beneath a pine tree in the enclosed circle made by its drooping lower branches, so like favorite places in our own neighborhood. Brown needles created a prickly mat, and the familiar scent, a blending of the fresh and dry needles, comforted me. As the afternoon went on, my grandparents were inside with Mother, while outside, taking turns guarding us were Maurine's cousin Katherine Donald and her mother, Sarah Donald. Kenny stabbed the toe of his shoe into the layer of pine needles, digging for the dirt beneath. I hung from my arms on a low, iron railing that lined a walkway of the hospital, next to the pine tree. The pipe was just high enough so that I could swing with my arms outstretched and not drag my bottom. Slowly I rocked back and forth, bending my knees, shifting from the heels to the toes of my white sandals, stirring the dust with my skirt, waiting for something to happen.

I remember all that—the hospital tree, its needles, my swinging, the hours of waiting, a picket for my fence.

WHEN, FINALLY, A WEEK OR SO LATER, the hospital released Mother, an ambulance carried her on the last leg of her long journey home. Accompanied by Maurine, she rode northwest along the rolling golden mesas at the base of the Rocky Mountains toward Boulder, then a university town of thirty thousand people, settled into and among the rocks and evergreens. As the ambulance crested a rise just outside the town, Mother spotted the Flatirons, enormous slabs of sandstone turned to vertical when the mountains heaved out of the earth to divide the continent. My grandmother said that when Mother saw the distinctive red rocks lying against the mountains, standing guard over the town, she wept. The sight told Mother she was home. Perhaps, it told her, too, there was something that hadn't changed.

A brick house on Tenth Street, around the corner, but sharing backyard space with my grandparents' house on College Avenue, waited for her. The Duhons, who had become close friends to my grandparents, had lived in that house until moving to a bigger one they'd built a few blocks away. The owner, another friend, rented the house to my grandparents when news came that Mother was returning. The location was ideal, close to Maurine and Hayes and to Aunt Lourie, who lived on the corner between us. Mother and Helen Duhon used to sunbathe on the flat roof of Aunt Lourie's garage overlooking the backyards while we children played below. But, of course, there was to be none of that in this edition of life in Boulder.

Our house was a single-story bungalow with a sunny dining room, which became Mother's room. From her rocking bed, she could see straight ahead through a wide doorway into the kitchen, to one side out the south-facing window and to the other into the living room. The bed, centered in the room, took up most of the space, but other equipment, all provided by the NFIP, crowded in, too. Her reclining wheelchair, a chest respirator, and a small end table for her suction machine stood by.

Four years ago, with my husband and son, I moved from the house where the airplane crashed in the backyard to a bigger one, with space for us and for the second child we were planning. This house, where I'm now firmly rooted, is just a couple of blocks up the hill from that rented one on Tenth Street. I often walk to the corner anchored by the three houses in which my family lived then. Many times I've gone slowly up the alley, trying to see it all as it was before fences, decks, and carports filled in the backyards. Other times, I end my early morning jog near the Tenth Street house so that I can notice how the morning light hits the dining-room windows in different seasons. I walk by, lingering on the sidewalk, thinking I might approach the front door and ask the people who live there now if I might look around inside. But I don't do it. I don't want to see it as it is now. I want to see it as it was *then*. I want those months I lived in that house with my mother to come into focus and roll like a movie before me, so I can inspect and relive it all. I want to remember what it was to live with my mother.

THE SUMMER OF 1955 PASSED QUIETLY for me. I often lay on the grassy mound that created a giant step between our house and the one next to us. Sometimes I rolled down the slope again and again, until I was sick to my stomach. Sometimes I lay with my head up and heels down and looked at the sky. Just outside Mother's window, it was a favorite place of mine. There I could be close to her, even see her if I stood atop the mound, and still be outside. On one particular day I lay there watching a strong, high wind move the clouds. I heard the neighbor's St. Bernard woof and considered going to visit him. A wooly brown-and-white bear of a dog, he was so gentle he let me ride him as if he were a pony. But I stayed where I was, seeing myself lying on my back: girl on summer afternoon, searching for familiar shapes in clouds. Another picket.

I can add a few more pickets to my fence from those peaceful summer afternoons when I explored a small section of our neighborhood. I walked the two-block stretch of College Avenue from our house to the College Grocery, run by Mr. and Mrs. Grant, at least once a day in the summer. I made my way there, sent by my grandmother to buy bologna by the slice for our lunch or by my grandfather for packages of Camel cigarettes. In the afternoon I went again for penny candy: cinnamon bears, candy corn, and licorice babies.

My grandfather was the mailman for our neighborhood, and each day I watched for him to come down the street at noon, his leather mail pouch slung over his shoulder. Margaret, a male bulldog with a brown eye patch who lived on the next corner with the Rook family, but who had free range of the neighborhood, often trotted along with Hayes and dropped by our house for a meal. I can still see Margaret, with his smashed-in face, standing at our back door, panting, blinking at us from those asymmetrical eyes, and waiting for our handouts.

Those summer months seemed tranquil to me, I suppose, because I had my mother back. The strangeness of our family life, with Mother paralyzed in the dining room and Dad nowhere in sight, isn't what impressed me; what did was that she was *there* again, talking to me and listening to me. In the way that all young children, I think, accept what is before them because they know no different, I didn't question the circumstances. It was enough that Mother had come back, however pale and small and unmoving she was in a giant bed that did move.

But for Mother and the other adults around us, that summer must have been anything but tranquil. For my grandmother, it couldn't have taken longer than a few hours for the pleasure of her daughter's return to be overshadowed by the reality of caring for someone who was helpless. Virginia had left three years earlier, a vibrant wife and healthy young mother, and returned in a state so dependent that she couldn't clear her own throat in the morning and needed her phlegm sucked out through a hole in her neck. I suppose the visiting nurses and someone from the local NFIP office could have showed them how to perform the necessary nursing duties; no doubt, however, there was a lot they had to figure out for themselves. And there was no one to help my grandparents with the personal alterations and adjustments they had to make in taking on the complex responsibility for their daughter's life. My grandmother was fifty-two when Virginia contracted polio. The long-established daily patterns of her life were turned upside down when Kenny and I were brought to Boulder to live with her and Hayes. And it doesn't take much to imagine the shock, a year after that, of Virginia's return. I know my grandparents loved their daughter and welcomed her back without reservation, whatever her condition. But love couldn't change the severity of the circumstances. Gone was the shared mother–daughter housewife camaraderie of the Maurine and Virginia from the before-Phoenix time—no more needlework or bridge games, no more baking and shopping together. I can only guess, with sadness, what these changes must have meant to each of them.

INSIDE THE FENCE I NOW TRY TO BUILD around this disturbing time are unanswered and unanswerable questions. And so I go back to building the fence: an accumulation of details and a chronology of events, if not explanation. I wanted to know what home life was like for Mother, beginning with her daily nursing and personal care. I questioned my father, Kenny, my grandmother, Katherine, neighbors and friends who knew us then. But I found that time and grief had erased the daily minutiae I wanted. To the few details I had, I added others taken from accounts of other quadriplegics and the family members who cared for them. And from that I've fashioned what I suppose was Mother's routine on Tenth Street.

What Maurine remembers most about Mother's care, or what she's most willing to tell me, is the suctioning. And that's how each day began, with removing the night's accumulation of Virginia's phlegm. The tracheotomy covering was slid open; a tube was inserted one to three inches; and the suction machine, the size of a small kitchen appliance, was flipped on to do its work. After all the careful efforts made at the Northwest Respirator Center to devise ways to make the suctioning as effective and unobtrusive as possible, Mother was now being drained by people who had none of that specialized experience.

Each morning someone gave Mother a bedpan, washed her face, made and fed her breakfast, gave her a sponge bath, rubbed her limbs with lotion, massaged her, and dressed her. She liked to have her hair combed and have lipstick applied. When I asked Ken for his memories, one detail he recalled was "lipstick on a glass straw," the kind once used in hospitals. It's an image, I, too, have carried. For many people, red lipstick evokes images of a womanly fifties mother applying her lipstick at a dressing table and leaving the outline of her lips on a highball glass, cigarette, or tissue. But we remember red lipstick on glass hospital straws.

What I learned from others who have cared for family members was that the morning routine could take three hours, completed in time to start lunch. Somewhere in each day, probably after lunch or in the evening, Mother was put into her wheelchair with the chest respirator, padded in all the sore spots it caused, and checked for proper function. Katherine remembers that Mother was most comfortable on the rocking bed, but that she used the wheelchair and respirator when she had company.

At night the routine was reversed. Mother was put back into the rocking bed, then onto the bedpan, was washed, and was dressed in her pajamas. Kenny remembers the cranks on the rocking bed, like any hospital bed, which moved the bed's head and foot. Those adjustments were done with some care and time in an effort to make Mother comfortable. She might have wanted a cushion under her knees, the sheet smoothed under her back, her clothing straightened. Any rumple would cause discomfort or pain long before the night was out.

Lou Sternburg had a buzzer rigged up on his bed so that he could summon his wife during the night to give him a sip of water, to move a leg, to scratch him, or to help him if he was choking "or in pain or afraid or lonely." And she was summoned ten or twelve times a night. I don't doubt the truthfulness of the Sternburgs' memoir, yet I can't envision how his wife kept up such a routine of devotion and sleep deprivation. Did she or he ever get an hour's uninterrupted sleep? I skimmed the surface of sleep through the nights of my sons' infancies, but I knew the drill was temporary. And maybe that's how Dorothy Sternburg and other caretakers did it, by telling themselves it wouldn't last forever.

Two nurses came in to help with my mother, though there's no doubt that Maurine bore the greatest weight for Mother's care. One nursing position was filled by a series of people who worked for a few weeks and then moved on, daunted, perhaps, by the magnitude of the caretaking the job required. The other was filled by a licensed practical nurse named Juanita Clark, who lived across the street. Nita, as we called her, was at our house part of most days caring for Mother, and because she couldn't resist children, she embraced Kenny and me as naturally as if we belonged to her. Although I last saw her decades ago, I can still picture her olive skin, tanned from hours in her garden, her two salt-and-pepper braids circling her head like a halo. When she wasn't at our house, Kenny and I sometimes crossed the street to visit her. In her dimly lit living-room she had a gumball machine welcoming Kenny and me and the many other children who visited often. Soft and kind, she laughed easily. I wish she were alive to give me her memories of what our life was like then.

No matter how much hired help is available, the relentlessness of the care that respiratory quadriplegics require wears on the primary caregiver. Betty Levin, whose husband, Alvin, came down with a severe case during the Boston epidemic of 1955, said that once in a while, through the years she lived with and cared for Alvin in their home, he would be hospitalized when a cold threatened to become pneumonia, and he'd sometimes stay an extra day or two to extend her rest. Going to bed without first getting someone else to bed, sleeping uninterrupted though the night, getting up in the morning, and dressing only herself were rare and appreciated reprieves from her daily and nightly routine. She had two extra respirators at home in case the one Alvin was using failed. She told me she'd sometimes wake in the middle of the night, hear the machine operating in an odd way, and get out of bed to check it, even before Alvin awakened. When I expressed to her my amazement over that nightly vigilance and the toll it must have taken, she said it didn't bother her. She raises sheep, she explained, and likens the care she gave her husband to being alert during lambing time, with an intercom in her bedroom linking her to the pregnant females. "I'm a shepherd," she explained.

Maurine was the shepherd in our house. In the weeks Dad stayed in Seattle, for job-related reasons, I suppose, she took charge of our household in Boulder. She slept on our living-room couch where she could see Mother and hear her bed moving. Mother's care became the focus of her life. Helen Duhon told me she watched with concern as Maurine lost weight and turned further inward. My grandmother had always been a worrier, but once she told me, as if confessing, that for all the disasters she had imagined and feared befalling her daughter, the one she had never given a thought was polio. Mother's condition, coupled with my grandmother's responsibility for her care, surely only intensified Maurine's conviction that disaster lurked around every corner. And in this situation, such vigilance was called for. Mother lived by machines, and machines can fail. In less time than it would take my grandmother to go home to her house across our small backyards to fetch a sweater or something from her refrigerator, Mother could be dead if she choked or if the machine she depended on to breathe broke down. She had perhaps four minutes to brain damage, six to death.

By THE TIME MY FATHER CAME TO JOIN US—and no one remembers just when that was, but perhaps before the summer was out—the patterns and routines of Mother's care had been established. There seemed to be no place for him, he said. "The fact is, I was still the outsider," he told me when I asked about what had happened during Mother's last months. "Things went downhill rapidly," he said. Living so close to in-laws probably would have been the right choice for most families, but not for ours, not for him.

Dad felt "forced" back to Boulder where he didn't want to be—forced, I suppose, by Mother, by Maurine and Hayes, by fate. Maybe he felt angry or guilty. Whatever the cause, the reformation of our family, with Dad at the head, never again came to be. Our family life had been mutating since the day she had gone into the hospital in Phoenix. By the time Dad tried to reenter in Colorado, something entirely different had taken its place. Maurine and Hayes were in charge. All attention focused on Mother. We children, I now think, were also incidental.

I'm not sure Dad was ever clear on what a father could or should do, having been reared without one himself. And certainly if he needed the cues of a "normal" family to tell him, he didn't have them in this alien setting. Perhaps he lost his sense of role, place, and purpose. Perhaps he felt inadequate to the task of caring for two children and an invalid wife; perhaps he felt as helpless as Mother was. Perhaps he just wanted out.

Trying to tell me how he saw the situation, how he felt, he said that he would come home from work, and Maurine and Hayes would "disappear." He would cook dinner and feed Mother and us children by himself. If he needed something at the grocery store, he'd have to get someone to watch us. Illustrating for me his misery at home, he told of the night Kenny had been sick and had vomited from his top bunk down into mine; when Dad had come in to clean up, he had vomited, too.

The weekends, Dad told me, were the worst because he "was a prisoner." Jack Clements told me that he didn't find care of his wife, Bette, difficult except for the confinement. A woman cared for Bette during the day while Jack went to work, but in the evenings and on weekends he was at home. He got haircuts and did other errands during weekday lunch hours. Groceries, as ordered by Bette on a speaker phone, were delivered to their house. In the evenings he and Bette watched television, had visitors, listened to jazz, and read and talked, in a routine that went on for a decade.

Dad, however, broke out of his "prison" within weeks by simply not coming home on weekends. That's when he learned to "oblivion drink," to block out his life, he said. His being away would upset Mother, and thus everyone in the family, he knew, but as he explained to me, he wasn't having fun either on those drunken weekends. Where he went, I don't know. A vagabond, he found women to drink with and sleep with. Again, offering explanation, he said: "I was twenty-nine and had needs." When he told me that, we were walking in the mountains, each of us with our eyes on the trail. Too stunned to react or notice whether his face was as casual and without regret as his words, I hiked on.

Surely Mother knew or at least suspected what he was up to. In their study of respiratory patients, the physicians Dane Prugh and Consuelo Tagiuri of Harvard Medical School and the Mary MacArthur Respirator Unit in Boston, found that a few "verbalized the fear of arousing resentment in husband or wife as a result of the demands of their illness, and it seemed very likely that they viewed abandonment as a possible consequence."

Dorothy Pallas, disabled with polio as a child, wrote as an adult of the fact of her dependency:

> To the severely handicapped, existence itself depends upon constant care. Sometimes we wonder if it is fair to impose this care on the people who happen to be near, family and friends. I have thought about this often and believe that just as our disabilities are circumstances of life which must be accepted if unchangeable, so the duty of caring for us is a circumstance of life to those on whom it falls. We should appreciate their help and give thanks for it but never waste our strength worrying about its fairness.

If Mother experienced similar fears of dependency and abandonment, they could only have deepened upon her "homecoming" when her fears came true: my father did abandon her, did betray her, did find her dependency too much to endure. My father, I fear, thought of fairness.

ONCE DAD BEGAN STAYING AWAY on weekends, Katherine and Sarah, Maurine's cousin and aunt, began coming from Denver to stay with us. Both of them humorous and warm people, they could turn any situation into an occasion just by showing up. They both told funny stories, and Aunt Sarah cooked hearty meals. Although Katherine is Maurine's first cousin, she's of my mother's generation, and she and Mother grew up together. They played as toddlers and children and later double-dated. Later still, Mother chose her to be my godmother. Sarah, who had been widowed young, and Katherine, who had not married, came not only to be company for Mother but to relieve Maurine.

When they came to visit, Katherine played Scrabble with Mother—they called each other "Kat" and "Virge"—and the two played other board games with us children, Mother bidding us to roll the dice for her and move her players. We gathered in the kitchen to fix dinner, in sight of Mother and often following her orders. One night she wanted "Coney Island hot dogs," made with pickle relish, mustard, and finely chopped onions. Katherine did the chopping and I carried them to Mother. "Not fine enough," she said, so I carried them back to Katherine for more chopping. One night Helen Duhon and Katherine decided to see who could hold a headstand the longest. Mother laughed so hard my grandmother had to stand by with the suction machine ready to drain the fluids from her throat. Together the women watched *The Perry Como Show* and *The Honeymooners* on television. Later, when the grown-ups continued watching television, and Kenny and I had been sent to bed, we would listen from our bunk beds, on the other side of the wall.

Most of these memories, these scenes of ordinary life, came to me from Katherine, who still lives in Denver. In recent years, I've asked her to tell me the stories more than once. Jackie Gleason and chopped onions on hot dogs became pickets for my fence, as well as reassurance for me that Mother—and I, too—had a sometimes happy home life with its simple, everyday pleasures. Reading an essay by Doris Lorenzen, paralyzed fully from polio in the 1920s at age eight, I was struck by one of her observations: "Normally endowed people claim they need an escape from reality; the severely handicapped person knows with passionate certainty that the wish to be a part of life is the only ambition that makes any sense."

Katherine's stories offer me views of my mother and her life that otherwise would be lost to me. In her affectionate shaping of the anecdotes I also can see myself as a child who had a mother and who was loved by her and others. Once, when I asked, she wrote a letter giving me some memories and told of preparing Thanksgiving dinner at her house the year Mother was in Seattle. All the women—Katherine, Sarah, Maurine, and my great-grandmother—were wrapped in aprons as they hustled around the kitchen. "You wanted a job, too," she wrote, "and so we trusted you with the silverware." But before I got to work, I demanded an apron like the others. "Where,"

Katherine wrote, "does one find an apron for a tiny fairy? Aunt Sarah tied a tea towel around you, and everyone got back to work."

Two other stories involve my mother directly, and so I treasure them even more. I don't remember either one, but I've taken them in as my own. Katherine tells of the day Mother asked her to give me a Toni permanent. Apparently I was pleased at the prospect of looking like Shirley Temple, but the procedure tried my five-year-old patience, and Mother and Katherine couldn't settle me. Then Dad passed by and remarked that I had pretty hair. As Katherine remembers it, I was so thrilled with the compliment that I cooperated from then on. Another time when Katherine was visiting, I went out to play with a friend, and Mother told me to be home at a certain time. Shortly past that time, I rushed in breathless and sweating, apologizing for my tardiness with, "I was saying 'Hail Marys' all the way home." These tales make me smile, and I enjoy hearing Katherine's fondness in the telling, but I can't help wondering about that little girl. Did I know how fragile Mother was, how tentative her existence? My guess is that I did not.

I don't know where in time to place the stories Katherine told me. The months Mother rocked in our dining room blur and blend, the days as indistinct as I suppose Mother's were from one another. What she did between the visits from Katherine and Sarah, I don't know, and no one can tell me. The weekends with the cadre of sociable women must have been the happy times. Katherine says she never saw my mother cry, but she also didn't see my mother during the in-between times, the long afternoons, the dark nights. My grandmother, who did, told me of just once seeing Mother's tears. It was when Father Charles Forsyth, a Benedictine priest widely loved in his parish, came to visit. Father Charles, who had lost a leg in World War II and walked with a cane or crutches, had come to our house before, but on that afternoon Maurine left the two of them alone. When she later returned, she saw they were both crying. Of the many scenes from my mother's life I wish I could have been privy to, that visit between Father Charles and Mother is near the top of the list.

My father tells me that one rare time when he and Mother spoke of what had happened to her, she said she thought polio was

God's punishment. As did many others, she thought she had done something to bring polio on. I wonder whether she told Father Charles, that day, her secret shames. And I wonder whether talking to him helped.

THE SUMMER PASSED, and then the fall, the measure kept by the whooshing of the chest respirator and the mesmerizing creaks of the rocking bed; from anywhere in our small house one could hear the humming, mechanical sounds of Mother being breathed. These were reassuring, lulling sounds. We became unaccustomed to silence, which was a signal for alarm. A fear of death, which no one spoke of, shadowed those months. Trouble could come at any moment. When Denverite Mary Leonard brought her polio-crippled husband home, she knew any disaster could occur, beginning with one of her nine children accidentally pulling the plug on her husband's breathers. When she brought him home, first in an iron lung, she said a prayer: "God, I'll do my best and do all I can, but I know that I can't do much so you'll have to do the rest." It was a prayer anyone in our household could have sent up to heaven, for we lived as if we knew we could do little, as if waiting for trouble. Mother was like a bubble we tiptoed around, fearing the worst. Often enough, something would happen to remind us of how fragile her existence was.

One weekend night, one of those nights when Dad was gone, Katherine slept on our living-room couch, while Sarah stayed next door at Maurine and Hayes's. In the early morning, Katherine, who must have been sleeping lightly, heard the rocking bed begin to slow and then stop. She rushed across the room to Mother and hollered at Kenny to run get Maurine and Hayes. She grabbed the portable respirator, which could be worked with a hand pump, and raised it high to fling it over Mother's chest. Mother's eyes, Katherine says, were wide, not so much with fright as with surprise at the sight of Katherine about to slam down a chest shell on her. And just then the bed went back on. A brief electrical outage had sapped its power.

Another evening, at about 8:00 or 9:00 P.M., Dad and Nita were with Mother, getting her ready for bed, when the house went black. The rocking bed stopped, and Mother was without air. Dad and Nita in their panic struggled with each other over Mother's body in the dark while trying to get the chest piece on her. Dad shouted orders as he secured the respirator and began pumping it. Kenny jumped down from his bunk and opened the door to the living room, where he saw flashlights moving back and forth, heard Mother sucking deep, gasping breaths, and heard Dad's frightening shouts. Ken ran to Maurine and Hayes's house, and Hayes rushed into our basement and replaced a blown fuse. As suddenly as it had started, the episode was over. The bed began rocking, Mother began breathing regularly, and the tension in our house edged up another notch.

I remember none of the episodes, and I may have slept through them, but the second power failure remains whole and horrific in my brother's memory. According to my grandmother, he seldom slept well and was particularly anxious on the nights when Dad wasn't home. One of those times, when Maurine slept in the guest guardian's place in our living room, she woke to find Kenny on Mother's bed, rocking with her. He said he thought he had heard her clicking for help.

We children were forbidden to get on Mother's bed. Maurine had made this rule not to protect us from falling off or getting caught under its powerful swing, which I've learned were reasonable cautions, but to protect Mother from our carelessness. Other children, some as young as Kenny and I, not only were allowed to get in bed with their handicapped parents, but also were involved in their care. I read of a four-year-old who learned to adjust her father's respirator and her six-year-old brother who could put it on him. "They love to help," their mother said at the time, noting that the children gave their father sips of water, moved his legs, and scratched his nose. Kenny thinks he might have helped feed Mother sometimes, because he remembers a time when she caught him staring at her tracheotomy hole and asked him what he was looking at. "There are crumbs on your neck," he said, but he refused to brush them away, for the tracheotomy frightened him.

One mother who feared that her young children would fall off the rocking bed or get crushed under it stationed a piano bench at the foot of the bed so the children could stand there to talk to their father. I picture Mother watching me and Kenny from her bed, from which we were warned to stay away, and think of the dozens of times and ways throughout a day that I touch my children. I know their bodies, those boys who are just out of babyhood, as well as my own. I can tell when they're ill by the change in their smells. I know where to kiss them to make them snuggle into me and where to kiss to make them laugh. When they cry, they wipe their eyes and noses and mouths on my chest and shoulder. If one were to devise a torture especially for mothers, it would be what my mother suffered: Look at your children, but don't touch them.

Recently, I was given cause to consider the touching that Mother and I missed when I was reunited with someone I'd long forgotten, someone whom I hadn't seen nor heard word of since the late fifties when we both left Boulder. She found me through an article I'd written for a magazine and left a message on my telephone answering machine. "Hello, this is Sister Mary David Terese," she said in a pleasant, somewhat excited voice. "I read your article and would love to talk to you. I don't know whether you remember me, but I just *know* you're the Kathy Black I once knew. I was your first-grade teacher." I dropped the mail I was sorting and played the message over and over, copying down and then rechecking the telephone numbers she gave. *Sister Mary David Terese.* I couldn't picture her face. My years at Sacred Heart, kindergarten through the middle of third grade, were a blur. I couldn't recall any of the nuns specifically, but she remembered me. I was one of hundreds of children Marie Greaney, who's still a nun but who now uses her original name, taught over the years, and yet she remembered specific contacts we had had.

I called her back, and she related for me a memory she had of our relationship, thirty-seven years past. She told me she used to comb my hair each day at school because she felt so sad that my mother couldn't touch me. Her own mother was "a wonderfully touchy person" who hugged and kissed her children freely, and the young nun knew what I missed by not having a mother to caress me. And so, each day, either at her desk or in the wood-paneled cloakroom, she brushed my hair, and we talked, before school, at lunchtime, and after school. I listened to this tender story and kept apologizing for not remembering her, trying to express my gratitude and trying to tell her my forgetting didn't mean it wasn't important to me. "It's okay," she reassured me, "you thanked me every day."

Hearing from her after so long an absence seemed a blessing on my search for my mother and the past. Sister Marie walked back into my life bearing more pickets for my fence. Hearing her memories helped me look back into that time and see how others around our family suffered, watching, imagining, being aware of my brother's and my circumstances and pain in a way we, as children, could not. And I saw, too, how my mind had closed out memories that could have comforted me, as well as those of fear and grief.

Sister Marie came to visit in person recently, and by talking of our time together, I've pieced together a sketchy picture of my first-grade year, that year Mother lived in our dining room. Kenny was in third grade then, and both of us remember that someone had attached a bulletin board to the wall next to the head of Mother's bed, and there, each day, we came home from school and eagerly thumbtacked our papers for her to see.

Draped in her order's layers of black serge and teaching her inaugural class, Sister Marie had sixty-three children in that first grade, nine of them named Michael. I suppose the only thing that made possible containing that many six-year-olds in one room was that we kept to our seats in orderly rows facing her big desk. Our huge room in the half-basement was bright with light from high sidewalk-level windows. My distinctions were that I was one of the smallest and youngest in the classroom, and my mother was paralyzed with polio, though no one spoke of her.

While I don't remember Sister Marie or her solicitude, one image of Sacred Heart has stayed with me through the years: two nearly life-sized statues that used to stand guard at the school's entrance. We children walked between them each day as we entered and departed. One was a robed, barefoot, long-haired Jesus with his hands raised in blessing. The other was an angel, not Gabriel, but a woman angel, a mother perhaps, with one arm around a waist-high girl. Her other arm was raised as if in greeting, and behind her, her grand wings, folded, swept to the ground.

DESPITE THE MANY KINDNESSES of Sister Marie and unnamed others, along with the jolly times engineered by Katherine and Aunt Sarah, our family was falling apart. I can't precisely place in time many of the details and memories I recall or have been told, but I can roughly order them by the slow, inexorable dissolution of our family as the months passed. Powerful emotion eddied around us: grief, sadness, fear. One of Kenny's former playmates told me he was afraid to come in our house. A girl my age who used to come seeking Nita's company, not mine, remembers being afraid in our house, too. She guessed the fear was a general one of illness and infirmity, but also specifically of polio. *Do you want to spend the rest of your life in an iron lung?* The image parents conjured for their children to keep them away from swimming pools and summer birthday parties lived in our house.

How did other families with similarly handicapped members manage to keep the fear and sadness at bay and hold themselves together? Those who coped better, I have decided, were the ones who tried to normalize their family life. I've been amazed to learn that some other families with a parent as handicapped as my mother went out into the world. They went to restaurants, stores, concerts, and church, and even on vacations, with the help of portable respirators, wheelchairs, slings, and lifts. In Seattle, Chancy Grace told me that although she often chafed, her parents, Hank and Janet Steputis, had approached obstacles cheerfully. If they had to enter a restaurant by the back door to get in with her father's wheelchair, for example, her mother might say brightly, "Gee, not everyone gets to see the inside of the kitchen." My mother, however, once she moved into our house on Tenth Street, never left it. Not once. Of her husband's return home, Dorothy Sternburg wrote: "I didn't want any of us to be ashamed of the way we lived or isolated by fear of what other people thought. I wanted our home to be approachable by everyone, not just pointed out as the house where the man on the rocking bed lived." But we were just that: the house where the woman on the rocking bed lived.

I think we could not find a way to make this transformed life normal for us, and so we withdrew from the larger world. According to Eric Cassell, chronically ill people, and by extension severely handicapped people, "despite . . . occasional expressions of unfairness, and attempts to hide, withdraw, or pretend indifference . . . try to stick it out in the world. They must remain part of the community; they need friends and associates, to have conversations, to achieve—they need all the things the rest of us require from group life." What families like the Sternburgs and Steputises were doing was giving their disabled members a place in the larger world. The emotional and physical risks were not great enough to cause them to withdraw from what Cassell calls "the ineluctable forces of human society."

On rare occasions, Mother was put in her wheelchair and taken out to our back patio. But our house had a short flight of stairs going to the backyard, so even that would have been a difficult task. A long flight from the front porch to the sidewalk would have prevented any exit for her out the front door. When confirming what I remembered about Mother never leaving the house, my father explained that it was "such a cumbersome process" with all the equipment that he couldn't do it alone. Not only that, he said, he didn't "enjoy being a spectacle." When he was out on his own in town, he said, he was embarrassed when people saw him on the street and said to him, "Oh my God, I heard what happened." To be out with Mother would have drawn more attention to himself than he could have tolerated. Besides, he said, "she didn't want to go out." I wonder whether that is so. How could she have not wanted to go out, even for a trip around the block? I read of one woman, similarly disabled, whose husband took her for walks in the neighborhood. She could breathe a bit on her own, but when she got tired, he tilted her wheelchair up and down to mimic the motion of the rocking bed. Maybe my mother, who could not breathe at all without a machine, was too full of fear to go out.

What society Mother had, came to her. My grandmother remembers that people visited "a lot"; my father says "no one visited."

And I doubt either is right. Dad wasn't there to know who was visiting, but I imagine few came during the times he was there. Dad says Mother was uncomfortable and that made others uncomfortable, but I suspect he was the most uncomfortable of all. And my grandparents were shy and not given to extending themselves into unknown social situations. Maurine and Hayes had their circle of friends and relatives among whom they could be lively and friendly, but they were never, as far as I can tell, widely social or involved in the community. So I doubt "a lot" of people came—uninvited or invited—to our house. Mary Sue Miles, the older sister of my best friend, Stevie, who lived at the top of our alley, told me she never once saw my mother. She knew she was there, but she never saw her.

As best I can tell, the rehabilitation begun at the Northwest Respirator Center stopped once Mother came home. I don't think she even continued with a low-calcium diet, since my grandmother remembers that Mother ate what the rest of us ate, apparently without any special diet. Mother also lost the skills she'd gained in Seattle. She no longer typed or even turned pages of books with a mouthpiece. No progress was made with her equipment either. In "The Vital Capacitor" newsletter, I read the accounts of the ongoing progress of discharged patients. One man, an engineer, as severely paralyzed as Mother, designed for himself two wheelchairs, one with a reading rack, food tray, and a place at the back for a respirator and another with retractable wheels to get him into a car. He also designed a hoist with four straps that went under his body to lift him from the wheelchair to his bed and back. Another motor-driven lift picked him and the wheelchair up as a unit and put them in a car. I searched issues of "The Vital Capacitor" published after Mother's discharge for news of her, but found only one sentence saying she was at home in Boulder with her children and husband. I suppose the issues were mailed to her, and I wonder what she thought when she read first that her friend Marylin Angell was free of respiratory aid, then that she was able to spend increasing periods of time on her feet, out of the wheelchair, and later that she was named New Mexico's polio mother of the year in 1956. There was no news of Mother, I suspect, because there was no progress. The newsletter didn't, understandably, include stories about patients who failed to progress at home, let alone those who declined. Mother's regression surely reflected the embattled emotional condition of our family. We weren't a team working toward common goals. My grandparents, who set the tone in our house, couldn't look too far into the future. And it seems that Dad wasn't much help in any way.

Despite our small circle of regular visitors, I wonder whether Mother felt more isolated than she had in Seattle. Did she miss the camaraderie of the respirator ward? Did being home in her condition take her to a new level of both understanding and distress? Again and again I've gone to Cassell's *The Nature of Suffering*, trying to reach my mother through her pain. Cassell enumerated what causes suffering, saying first that it is individual. He continued:

> We all recognize certain injuries that almost invariably cause suffering: the death or suffering of loved ones, powerlessness, helplessness, hopelessness, torture, the loss of a life's work, deep betrayal, physical agony, isolation, homelessness, memory failure, and unremitting fear. Each is both universal and individual. Each touches features common to us all, yet each contains features that must be defined in terms of a specific person at a specific time.

I read that list and check all those that Mother endured, many of them at the same time, and wonder whether there is a limit to what a person can bear. Her physical pain went on in the form of sensitivity, aching muscles, stiff joints, indigestion, and kidney stones. And the mental anguish was unremitting as well, not only for her but for those of us around her. My brother, who slept fitfully at home, threw up at school. I tried to be a good girl and stay out of the way. Dad was gone more and more often, disappearing for days when he got a paycheck, sometimes not coming home even during the week. My grandmother tells the story of him returning one Friday evening after an absence of some days and hearing my mother say: "He's come home just in time to spoil my weekend."

MARCELLE DUNNING TOLD ME that when Mother was discharged from the Seattle center, she had grasped the concept that she was going to have to live with her handicap. But she also told me that many people go home hoping for a miracle, which wasn't a bad strategy, for "if you can't have that, you go home without much." Lou Sternburg wrote that even after he moved back home, he kept up hope, even the expectation, that his situation would somehow change. "A new therapy would be discovered, a new cure," he thought. That belief, he said, "kept me going and made me able to live with the pain." He added: "There is no doubt that maintaining the endless illusion that I would walk again was one of my strongest weapons for survival." I know that my grandmother nurtured the same belief about my mother, for one of the few stories she ever told me during my childhood about my mother was that soon after she came home, Mother discovered she could wiggle a foot. Maurine always told this story wistfully, implying that walking and breathing could not have been far behind. Mother didn't share that thinking, according to Katherine, who remembers being excited when Maurine and Hayes told her of this new development. Katherine went eagerly to Mother saying she'd heard the great news. And Mother replied: "It's nothing, just a nerve twitching." Katherine persisted: "Well, that's good if there's a nerve there. Maybe we should rub it or something." And Mother simply said: "No." Katherine said she went on hoping, as "it was hard not to." This anecdote makes me wonder again whether Mother's internal regulator, the psychological mechanism that keeps the truth from overwhelming people, didn't function well for her. Could she see too clearly her condition? Was hope in too short supply in our home?

My grandmother kept a tiny vial of an oil that flows from the relics of Saint Walburga, a venerated saint of medieval Germany. A small group of Benedictine nuns came to Boulder from Germany as political refugees in the 1930s and established an abbey in the name of Saint Walburga east of Boulder. They farmed the land, selling milk from their cows and eggs from their chickens, and they prayed and dispensed, at special request, drops of the precious healing oil they had brought from their motherhouse in Eichstätt, Germany. I know we had the oil, which Maurine kept cushioned in cotton in a jewelry box. I don't know whether or how it was used on Mother or what powers it was expected to have. My grandmother, I think, prayed for a miracle, but she also prayed to Saint Jude, one of the twelve apostles and the patron saint of desperate, if not lost, causes.

I GATHER UP THE FEW REMAINING PICKETS and add them to my fence. One is a small pile of undated photographs I have from my early childhood. In there is a picture of a tumbleweed sprayed with artificial snow and decorated with glass balls. We had a tumbleweed like that in Arizona for a Christmas tree, but this photograph was taken in Colorado. I know because Aunt Sarah is in the picture, and she never visited us in Arizona. I suppose that picture is from Christmas of 1955, the year Mother came home to us. But it strikes me as peculiar today. Who would want a tumbleweed for a Christmas tree in a home resting among evergreens? And how did it get to Colorado? But like so much else in our life then, to my child's eyes it was accepted as the way we did things.

When Ken and I had our first deliberate conversation about our mother's illness and death, thirty-five years after her funeral, he spoke of the memories as an iceberg beginning to move inside him as we talked. He remembered the tumbleweed Christmas tree, but nothing else about that Christmas. He was eight then, but his memory is as wounded as mine. He says it's as if we didn't celebrate Christmas at all that year. I don't remember anything of it either, but I do have a strong memory of my birthday, my sixth, which came right before.

On that day I was ordered to close my eyes and await a big surprise. I stood in our living room, surrounded by adults, my eyes squeezed closed. Maurine and Hayes, Katherine and Aunt Sarah, my great-grandparents, and Mother in her wheelchair formed a semicircle behind me. Kenny must have been there, too, and maybe even Dad, but I don't remember. I was instructed to open my eyes, and there before me was the most beautiful doll I'd seen in all my six years. She was sitting in a child-sized maple rocking chair. The doll, with a porcelain head, eyes that opened and closed, and real hair on her head, was almost as big as I was. I kept silent, unable to express the joy I felt, overwhelmed by the present. The doll was old, having been given first by my great-grandmother to my grandmother, who had given it to Mother, who was now giving it to me. In some intuitive way of a young girl, I understood the magnitude of this gift, the connection it gave me to my mother, my grandmother, my great-grandmother, the women behind me in the room and in time. The rocker was new, selected especially for me. The decision to give those treasures to me that birthday, Katherine tells me, was made and planned with great excitement by my mother.

In later years I always played with the doll alone, never sharing her with my friends. And I never gave her a name. I know I associated her with my mother. The doll came to me wearing a 1920s-style flapper dress of a wispy red fabric, decorated with red ribbon. It couldn't have been the doll's original outfit, for she had been given to my grandmother at the turn of the century, but it must have been a dress my mother had gotten for her. She also wore a crocheted ecru cap and sweater, tied with pink ribbon woven through crocheted loops, which my mother had worn as a baby. On her feet were a pair of tiny, white leather button shoes that had been worn on my grandmother's baby feet. I also had an ivory-handled button hook that was my grandmother's. I hooked and unhooked those shoes endlessly. Although I tried to be careful, I couldn't resist the doll, and over time, I painted her fingernails red and combed her soft brown hair until it was matted and thin.

MY LAST TWO MEMORIES ARE DISTURBING ONES. They are not unlike those every child must harbor, but in the sparsity of my remembered past, they rise in unnatural relief. In them both, Mother is angry with me. The first came when I got a new pair of black patent leather shoes, and like so many other of my memories, I don't know where to put the vivid scene in time, but I think it came after Christmas. Mother was in her usual place in the dining room, watching and listening, while a group of women gathered in the kitchen talking. Wearing my new shoes, I gravitated toward them and began tap dancing, enjoying the *rat-a-tat-tat* sound the crisp leather soles made on the kitchen floor. Paying no attention to the women and their conversation, but wanting to be in their company, I tapped and tapped, doing my best Shirley Temple imitation, feeling talented, imagining myself performing on-stage. Suddenly my mother's voice, sharp and angry, called out to me: "Kathy! Stop it! Stop that noise!" I froze. Not once since Mother had become ill had she talked harshly to me. I fled to my bedroom, terror, indignation, and confusion ricocheting in me. Rather than face Mother again after such humiliation, I decided to run away. I pulled out my red suitcase, a cosmetic case handed down from Maurine, and packed it with a pair of pajamas and as many toys as would fit. And I went out the back door.

I stood in the backyard, silent houses in the late afternoon offering no direction. Almost every house in our neighborhood had a front porch, but the action took place in the backyards and in the alley, anchored at one end by us and at the other by the Miles family, where the two youngest boys, Danny and Stevie, were best friends to Kenny and me. On that late afternoon, however, no one was there, only the fading light as the sun dropped behind the mountains. My indignation and sorrow spent, I could think of nowhere to go except to my grandparents' house, just steps away. I walked in their back door and found my grandfather there. I carried my suitcase to the basement, where my grandmother hung the laundry to dry on Mondays, and lay down on an old spare bed. I don't know what I hoped for or wanted, but my humiliation was complete when my grandmother returned from our house and told me she and my grandfather were going back there for dinner, and I might as well come, too.

The second memory dates to Easter that year, which fell on April 1. Mother had asked Katherine to buy a new Easter dress for me, and Easter bunnies, stuffed toy ones, for Kenny and me. When Mother presented the rabbits to us, one lavender, one yellow, she and Kenny agreed that I could take my pick. For reasons I can't explain, their generosity overwhelmed me. Maybe I wanted to test their love. Perhaps it was simple immaturity and lack of confidence in my ability to choose and be happy with my choice. Whatever it was, I couldn't decide. First I took the lavender one, but as soon as Kenny picked up the yellow bunny, its appeal was too great for me to resist, and I asked for it instead. But again I wavered when I saw the lavender one in his arms; lavender was my favorite color. Mother and Kenny put up with this through another change of mind, and then, exasperated, Mother told Kenny to take one and let me have what was left. I suppose to almost any other child such a scene would be lost in the layer on layer of memories, happy and sad, angry and loving, between mother and child that went on over the years. But for me, those two memories hovered over the next decades of my life. They were my last memories of Mother.

CHAPTER EIGHT

Answered Prayers

While my mother rocked in our dining room and our family, isolated by fear and circumstances, sank deeper into the world of polio, the nation concluded its obsession with the disease. The country's long quest for deliverance from polio, begun early in the twentieth century, ended by the spring of 1956.

Long before there was a National Foundation for Infantile Paralysis funding research efforts, scientists had zealously, relentlessly, and unsuccessfully pursued an end to the crippling disease. Through the decades, while scientists struggled to understand polio, its destruction spread. In 1931 an epidemic almost as bad as the one in 1916 hit the northeastern United States. Philadelphia was besieged in 1932, Los Angeles in 1934, New York in 1939, and Huntington, West Virginia, in 1941. And the worst epidemic years were yet to come.

Scientists faced formidable obstacles in unlocking the secrets to polio's nature. After first hunting for a polio bacteria, researchers determined in 1908 that it was a viral disease, which made understanding how it behaved in the body only more difficult. Once researchers isolated the virus, they were further hindered by the fact that the only other creature susceptible to the disease was the monkey, which posed practical limitations on researchers. Scientists were further hampered by the fact that no one knew the true incidence of polio, because most cases were inapparent. That made the disease impossible to avoid, and all efforts to cure it had led to dead-ends. Thus, immunization seemed the most likely source of salvation, but even after decades of research, hopes for a vaccine continued to be dim.

Part of the reason was that doctors, scientists, and public health officials were frightened at the thought of vaccinating against polio. In the early forties it was known that the vaccines that work best against viruses contained the live virus, which always carried a risk of infection, but fresh in the minds of anyone who might have wanted to pursue that solution was the tragic summer of 1935. Two different live polio vaccines tested then infected children with the disease rather than protected them; some died.

Scientists considered the safe option of passive immunization, the injection either of blood carrying antibodies or of gamma globulin, a blood protein that acts as an antibody. In the early fifties, with an NFIP grant, William McDowell Hammon, a physician at the University of Pittsburgh, directed gamma globulin studies to see what protection from polio could be provided. Injections given over two summers showed that the extract did give short-term immunity. In his report in the *Journal of the American Medical Association*, however, Hammon wrote that gamma globulin was an impracticable means of polio prevention, because of its cost and incompleteness of protection. "Immunity is high for five weeks," he wrote, "drops off during the next two, and disappears after eight weeks." Hammon had, however, shown that antibodies could provide at least short-term protection against paralytic polio, a finding that helped renew the quest for vaccination.

The public, however, grasped in the gamma globulin research what they wanted to hear—news that something was being done, that they were not helpless against polio. Mothers and fathers learned that gamma globulin was a polio-protector, and they wanted it, demanded it. The NFIP, despite what it knew about the cost and shortage and relative uselessness of gamma globulin distributed on a mass scale, wanted to give the public what it wanted. The government had classified the material as strategic and controlled the supply, but the persuasive NFIP leader Basil O'Connor talked the Department of Defense into turning it over. People from public health services tried to dissuade him, citing bad epidemiology and a waste of important supplies. But O'Connor persisted, and in 1953 the NFIP bought the nation's entire supply for $5.5 million.

For the public, that five or seven weeks' protection was better than nothing. It might mean getting a child through the worst of a polio season or a session at summer camp, and to mothers of children with polio it could give assurances about the safety of healthy siblings. Around the country, parents like those of Roger Beck, an eight-year-old boy living in Minnesota in the summer of 1953, calmed their fears by getting the injections (delivered with very large needles) for their children. Beck's parents were "well-educated, well-traveled people not given to alarm," he says, but when he came down with a high fever that lasted just a day, his parents took no chances and ordered gamma globulin for all their children.

Communities set up clinics to deliver free gamma globulin shots to schoolchildren. Others dispatched them to children headed for summer camps. When a hospital worker came down with polio, the whole staff was inoculated. In Pitman, New Jersey, four cases were reported within a week in the fall of 1954, and the town mobilized to deliver gamma globulin to children and expectant mothers. Mass inoculations started on a Saturday night, and 7 doctors, 5 dentists, 25 registered nurses, and 300 hastily mobilized volunteers injected 1,632 people in just seven hours. The *Arizona Republic*, reporting that free inoculations were available to children and camp counselors, called gamma globulin a "versatile serum," since it prevented not only polio but also measles and infectious hepatitis. "The amazing serum," the reporter called it, "helps relieve the worry parents feel for the health of their children during sessions at summer camp."

And all that effort went to waste. A committee of experts from the U.S. Public Health Service and the U.S. Department of Health, Education, and Welfare (HEW) evaluated gamma globulin data and found that the serum failed to halt the disease either by preventing cases or lessening the severity of the attack. The committee also concluded that "family contact" use (where the family members of polio cases are inoculated as soon as the illness is diagnosed) also did not reduce the number of cases.

AVOIDING POLIO, curing polio, injecting gamma globulin— none of it worked. What the country, the *world* needed was a safe and effective vaccine. As it turned out, not just one but two were on the way.

In the forties, many lab scientists labored at their benches pursuing vaccines with inactivated or killed viruses. Writing in *Harper's* in 1945, Howard A. Howe, the physician who headed the Poliomyelitis Research Center at Johns Hopkins University, said: "Perhaps some day we shall reach the goal by this route." He was right, but before an effective vaccine could be made, previously intractable questions had to be answered. First, how many types of polio virus existed? Answering that would require painstaking, time-consuming, expensive research. But it was just the sort of job the NFIP was ideally suited to handle. It stepped in both to fund and to direct a typing program, assigning the tedious work to virologists at several universities around the country. The task began in 1948 and ultimately used 17,500 monkeys and cost $1,190,000 before being completed in 1951. Jonas Salk, the physician who was the spokesman for the labs and then the director of the Virus Research Laboratory of the School of Medicine at the University of Pittsburgh, reported the results: three polio viruses had been identified. As many as 196 had been suspected, so this sorting into only three categories showed that the development of a vaccine would be less complex than some had thought.

The second important piece of the puzzle was placed in 1949 when the physician John F. Enders and his associates at the Harvard Medical School discovered that the polio virus could be grown in test-tube culture on monkey tissues of nonnervous origin. Until then, it was thought that the virus could grow only in the nerve tissues of humans and a few species of monkeys. Because vaccines prepared from nerve tissue carried a risk of causing brain damage to the recipient, the findings that nonnervous tissue could be used opened a way to a safe polio vaccine.

The final question was whether the virus entered the bloodstream before it attacked nerve cells. Since antibodies form in blood, it was unlikely that a vaccine would produce antibodies against a virus that bypassed the blood altogether. Dorothy M. Horstmann at Yale and David Bodian at Johns Hopkins independently succeeded in recovering virus from the blood of monkeys and chimps three to five days after the animals had been infected. At that news, excitement among scientists ran high.

Those and other discoveries led to a report given at a low-key meeting of the NFIP committee on immunization in Hershey, Pennsylvania, in January 1953. There, Salk informed other scientists that he had injected 161 human subjects with what he believed was an effective killed-virus polio vaccine. Appearing in the March 1953 issue of the *Journal of the American Medical Association*, Salk's article, "Studies in Human Subjects on Active Immunization against Polio-myelitis," provided the world with the first detailed report of his work.

By 1952, Salk had been satisfied he had a vaccine safe for humans, but that summer when *Life* quoted another scientist as saying it would be ten years before a vaccine could be made, he kept silent and went on with his work. He had developed a vaccine using viru-lent forms of polio that were then killed with formaldehyde and in-jected. The killed vaccine provoked the body's immune system into manufacturing antibodies that would fight the polio virus in the wild, should the person later encounter it. Injecting children, among them his own, with his vaccine took courage, he said, but it was courage that came from confidence based on experience, not daring. None-theless, he admitted that he did not administer the shots without emotion. "When you inoculate children with a polio vaccine," he said in a characteristic understatement, "you don't sleep well for two or three months."

Salk's 1953 announcement brought to a high pitch the long-held public hope and conviction that infantile paralysis would be conquered. It also spotlighted the long-awaited polio hero. Most may have missed his name when announcements were made about the typing of the virus, but once the vaccine news was out, Salk's name became permanently linked to polio.

Public enthusiasm and expectations put pressure on the NFIP, which had by choice become the focus of the fight against polio. For years, the NFIP had been able to use the compassion of the public to collect ever-larger amounts of money, but by the early fifties the pub-lic was impatient for results. They had poured an average of $25 million a year into the organization since 1938, and still the number of polio cases had continued to grow, reaching a frightening high of fifty-eight thousand in 1952. The NFIP was also feeling the pressure of its promise to pay for the care of the mounting rolls of polio patients. Despite its research goals, the care of patients always took most of the funds. Between 1938 and 1955 the NFIP spent almost ten times as much money on patient care as on research. The growing number of polio survivors was straining even the considerable fund-raising powers of the NFIP.

THE TIME HAD COME FOR A SOLUTION, and Salk seemed to have it. Before his vaccine could be licensed by the government, commercially manufactured, and injected into the arms of millions, though, it had to be tested. And on whom could the testing be done? Animals don't get the disease naturally, so all the laboratory tests on them—and there had been many—were of limited use. Adults who might have willingly volunteered likely already had antibodies to polio, having been exposed to the virus at some time in their lives. For scientists to know for sure whether Salk's vaccine, or any other, was both safe and effective, they needed a sampling of thousands of children, who could be inoculated and whose incidence of polio could then be compared to a control group of unvaccinated youngsters after the year's polio season had passed.

The NFIP, acting on the advice of a medical committee headed by the physician Tom Rivers, an advisor to the NFIP with the Rockefeller Institute, decided to fund such a field trial of Salk's vaccine, using the nation's first-, second-, and third-graders, the most polio-susceptible population group. By mid-November 1953 plans were in place to start inoculating children on February 8, 1954. But in the months before the trial could begin, doubts, compromises, second thoughts, and reformulated plans came from the scientific and medical communities, from government officials, from within the NFIP, and even from Salk.

February 8 came and went without a single child being inoculated, in part because the five drug companies producing the vaccine failed to deliver the needed doses. Some of the first batches were thrown out because tests showed they may have contained live virus. Debate went on in the public forum and privately in medical science circles about whether the NFIP and the government were moving too fast to ensure a safe vaccine. But the supporters persisted. If the injections were delayed too far into the spring of 1954, there would not be time to inoculate enough children to make the test meaningful before summer arrived. And the vaccine could not be administered once the polio season was under way, because then there would be no way to tell whether the year's cases were a result of the vaccine or not.

March passed. Then on April 4, 1954, a Sunday night, the trial efforts took a blow from the broadcaster Walter Winchell. Winchell's program, a combination of hard news, gossip, and opinion, had once reached two thirds of American adults through radio or newspaper syndication. By 1954 he was past that peak of popularity, but when he closed the first half of his newscast that night by saying, "In a few minutes I will report on a new polio vaccine announced as a polio cure. It may be a killer," the nation was listening. He came back on the air and said, "Attention all doctors and every family in the United States . . . " and reported, irresponsibly and untruthfully, that the U.S. Public Health Service had found that seven of ten batches of the Salk vaccine contained live polio virus. The NFIP quickly noted that only four lots had been thrown out and that finding them was the whole point of testing. Salk went public again to say that he had just given his own children booster shots of the vaccine.

The next Sunday, Winchell kept up his scare tactics and quoted the physician Albert B. Sabin, an eminent polio researcher at the University of Cincinnati College of Medicine, as saying he thought the tests should be delayed. A doctor at the Mayo Clinic was quoted as saying he would not give the vaccine to his children. Winchell further claimed that the NFIP was stockpiling little white coffins in depots around the country, so they would be ready for the children who were killed during the field trial. After the broadcasts, several cities and counties set up as trial sites backed out of the program. Jane S. Smith, author of *Patenting the Sun: Polio and the Salk Vaccine*, wrote:

To those who were making the decision, it still seemed possible that the entire trial might be postponed another year. There was little anybody could learn in another year that they didn't know already—little they could ever learn without the very field trial they were debating—but they were all made nervous by the accelerating rush of events. Up until the very last moment, the members of the Vaccine Advisory Committee still couldn't quite bring themselves to say the trial vaccine was safe to use. Neither could the director of the Laboratory of Biologics Control. The children were ready, the photographers had their flashbulbs in the sockets, the lollipops were waiting, the polio season was edging north, but the people making the decisions were scared. They were scared by Walter Winchell's little white coffins. They were scared by the virulent strains of virus Salk insisted on using in his vaccine. They were scared by Albert Sabin's eternal 'what ifs.' What if they gave the go-ahead and children started keeling over across the country? It was absolutely terrifying.

Nothing better illustrates both the fear polio instilled in parents of the early fifties and the faith they held in medical science than the fact that, by the tens of thousands, they signed the forms and marched their children forward for their shots once the trial did begin. Despite rumors about risks, despite what they might be able to imagine for themselves about the consequences, they lined up to get the unproved protection for their children. As Smith, a "polio pioneer" (as the children who participated in the trial were called), wrote: "In all the literature that surrounded the effort, the word 'permission' was never used. Neither were 'volunteer,' 'experimental,' or 'test.' Parents had to 'request' to 'participate' in a 'trial.' " And they did. Thousands of little vials labeled "Polio Vaccine, Types 1, 2 and 3, Caution: New Drug" were released into the hands of doctors, and at 9:00 A.M. on Monday, April 26, 1954, the designated first child,

Randy Kerr, age six, of Fairfax County, Virginia, was inoculated. In the next weeks, 650,000 children in forty-four states were administered three shots each. Of those, 440,000 received the actual vaccine, and the rest got a placebo. The Winchell broadcasts reduced the number of volunteers by about 10 percent, some said, but in the end, the 650,000 participants were enough.

A writer for the *New Yorker* visited Public School No. 61, on Manhattan's Lower East Side, to interview some little pioneers as they participated in the trial. First, some were given blood tests to determine whether they already had polio antigens in their blood. (Some of the children might have already had one or more of the three types of polio and thus would have been immune. Part of the trial involved computing the frequency of such cases.) After the blood test, each child was then led to another room to be "swabbed, jabbed, swabbed, and sent away with a quick pat on the back and a word of praise." The reporter struck up a conversation with a few of the third-graders:

> A dark-haired girl whose first name was Alida and whose last name was an Italian aria that we couldn't quite catch . . . had not minded the blood test. It had been worse than she had expected, but she had not *minded* it. The shot was going to be cinchy—just like a mosquito bite. One of the other kids had told her. After her shot, she was going back to her classroom for her regular midafternoon snack, which consisted of milk, a pretzel stick, and a cherry-cheese sandwich. . . . Next to Alida was a brown-faced boy named Jimmie. Jimmie wanted to make our flesh creep. "It wasn't how far in they stuck the needle, it was how long they left it there," he said with relish. Pamela, a seat beyond Jimmie, ordered him not to be a stupe. "Our teacher said we were pioneers," said Pamela. "Like the old pioneers, only not on land but in"—her eyes fell, and she pursued the forgotten word and found it—"knowledge." Susan and Harriet, seated beside Pamela, nodded. They were glad to be shot as pio-

neers. Did we understand, they asked, about vaccines? About controls? About immunity?

Children did not keel over by the thousands, the little white coffins never materialized, and the country sat back to await the tedious collection and tabulation of the results. Some people thought the answer—a positive one—came that fall when the NFIP committed $9 million to six drug companies to start stockpiling the Salk vaccine so that it would be ready for the spring of 1955. But that was not the case. The NFIP thought the vaccine was effective, or it would not have spent $7 million for the field trial. Like everyone else, however, it was awaiting news from physician Thomas Francis Jr., the director of the Poliomyelitis Vaccine Evaluation Center at the University of Michigan, who was charged with interpreting and reporting the results. Meanwhile, with the trial going on into the evaluation months of 1954, while the country crept toward its miracle, 38,500 Americans, my mother among them, came down with polio.

THE OFFICIAL REPORT coming from Dr. Francis was scheduled to be made public on April 12, 1955, the tenth anniversary of the death of Franklin D. Roosevelt. In the meantime, rumors circulated in newspapers about the results, and with each one Francis and the NFIP continued to say the data simply were not compiled yet. Polio, always news, was now constantly in the headlines. The nation—the world—was poised for a thumbs-up, but as the *New York Times* reported, "No top secret during the war has been more zealously guarded than the findings at the [evaluation] center."

Then on the morning of April 12 in Ann Arbor, Michigan, Francis, described by the *New York Times* as "a short, chunky man with a close-cropped mustache," wearing a "black suit, white shirt and striped gray tie," stood up before an audience of five hundred scientists and physicians and a battery of television, newsreel, and radio microphones and read his long-awaited report. The trial showed that the vaccine was effective and safe. Although he spoke in a "conversational tone," the moment was a dramatic one, according to a *New York*

Times reporter present at the University of Michigan campus for the announcement, "no matter how hard the Professor of Epidemiology tried to make it otherwise with his charts and statistics and careful qualifications."

Around the country people read and heard the news and rejoiced. "It's a great day. It's a wonderful day for the whole world," said Oveta Culp Hobby, the HEW secretary. An official from the American Medical Association called the report "more thrilling than any detective story." Eleanor Roosevelt placed a wreath on her husband's grave and then told reporters she was "delighted" with the outcome of the trial.

Across the country, reporters rushed with their microphones and notepads to the polio wards to do the irresistible feature story: What did those for whom the vaccine came too late think of the nation's big news?

For some, the news carried heartbreak. From her iron lung in the decrepit Kingston Avenue Hospital in New York City, nine-year-old Sharon Stern watched the news of the successful Salk vaccine on a television. The previous October, as data from the field trials were being collected, she had come down with a severe case of polio. After three nightmarish days and nights, she had become paralyzed from the neck down. When her mother came to visit that April 12, she sat at the head of Sharon's iron lung and wept. "Seven months," she said. "Couldn't you have waited seven months?"

Early that same morning print and broadcast reporters showed up at the Northwest Respirator Center in Seattle, where my mother lay, to interview patients there. A writer for the *Seattle Post-Intelligencer* said, "Word that the Salk vaccine has been proved successful was received joyfully in the sunny wards on the fourth floor of the hospital." He included a quote from Dorothy Baldwin, twenty-five, who said, "It came too late for me, but thank God it comes in time for my children!" She was, the reporter said, voicing "the feelings of thousands of persons who have been struck down by the disease." Photographs accompanying the front-page story showed a twenty-year-old woman in an iron lung, Baldwin in bed with photos of her children next to her, Lauretta Knutson weaving a place mat on a small bed loom, and twenty-one-year-old, dark-eyed Fred Lien lying on a bed and breathing with a chest respirator.

I searched the story for comments from my mother and found none. But later I read in an issue of "The Vital Capacitor" that cameras and reporters from KING-TV, a local television station, had interviewed patients the same morning. And the "stars" of the evening news report included Virginia Black. "What a performance!" wrote Jeanne Baldwin in "The Vital Capacitor." Someone had recorded my mother on film. The possibility that my mother's voice and animated face, lost to me forty years ago, were preserved on film was almost more than I could take in. I let weeks pass before I picked up the telephone and called KING-TV to ask what I needed to do to see the footage. I learned that the station had preserved nothing before 1965—not even footage about one of the decade's, maybe the century's, most important news stories.

Reports about the successful vaccine took on a euphoric cast. It was the kind of news that made writers let loose with effusions. In the *Minneapolis Morning Tribune*, the science writer Victor Cohn said: "The development of polio vaccines, present and future, is a monument to several important things. To initiative and individualism, and to willing cooperation. To the spirit of starting things, and of getting things done. To the American volunteer—'the guy who pitches in.' " He went on to call it a monument to "thousands of ordinary citizens—volunteer workers and givers—who have taken part in a movement unique in the world history, the mass movement started barely 20 years ago to defeat this disease." He was forgetting, perhaps, that the fight against polio was not born with the NFIP.

An editorial in the *New York Times* called the announcement "a turning point in medical history. Gone are the old helplessness, the fear of an invisible enemy, the frustration of physicians. Gone, too, are the 'iron lungs' in which the paralyzed languished, and gone the hot-weather epidemics of poliomyelitis. Science has enriched mankind with one of its finest gifts."

An important, vital step had been taken, but polio was not gone. Even as the news was reported, another polio season was getting under way. Twenty-nine thousand people contracted the disease in 1955, including almost four thousand in the Massachusetts epidemic that summer and fall. The irony of the timing of the Boston epidemic was not lost on the patients and doctors there, according to the physician William Tisdale, "A lot of patients or friends were either dead or extremely crippled," he told me, remembering that summer, "and they had missed the immunization boat."

JUST BEFORE MIDNIGHT ON APRIL 12, 1955, at the end of the history-making day, a 430-pound shipment of vaccine from the Cutter Laboratories in Berkeley, California, arrived by United Airlines in Seattle. A second shipment of 224 pounds came in by Northwest Airlines from Detroit for local Parke, Davis & Company offices to distribute. Rationing of these shipments and others around the country began immediately. Despite the early preparations and the $9 million of vaccine the NFIP had ordered, there would not be enough vaccine for everyone who wanted it that first spring. A spokesman for Cutter said that company could have sold its entire April allotment for the western part of Washington State to two pediatricians. "The vaccine will be scarcer than hen's teeth for a while," he said. Still, the day after the announcement in Ann Arbor, communities started inoculating children. Wherever the vaccine was available, parents with their children stood in lines that sometimes snaked for blocks around doctors' offices. Clinics stayed open late to accommodate everyone. Children filed into school gymnasiums reeking of rubbing alcohol to get their shots.

In the week following the Ann Arbor announcement, newspapers were peppered with jocular stories about the vaccine as it began to be administered. "PSYCHOLOGY GIVES WAY TO NICKEL," was the headline for a story out of Topeka where the famous psychologist Karl Menninger was helping to immunize grade-schoolers. It seems that one eight-year-old resisted all his psychological persuasion and refused the needle until Menninger reached into his pocket and drew out a coin to bribe the boy.

Each day Americans picked up their newspapers, flipped on their radios and televisions, and got the latest on the new vaccine. Much discussed was the price. The NFIP planned to give away its vaccine to first- and second-graders; while the rest of the nation's supply would be distributed through physicians. A spokesman for McKesson & Robbins, Inc., one of the wholesaler firms that would distribute the vaccine in the Seattle area, estimated that the cost for the three-shot series would be about $20 through private physicians. The next day the *Seattle Times* ran a story quoting doctors who said the estimate was about twice what they expected it to be. The New York State Health Commission put the price at $3.50, plus the physician's charge. A manufacturer put the cost at $6 for the three-shot dose, before the physician's fee.

The big news, however, continued to be the shortage. Only hours after the Ann Arbor announcement was made, the U.S. Public Health Service declared the vaccine safe and potent, and HEW's Oveta Culp Hobby extended licenses to six U.S. manufacturers to produce and distribute the vaccine. Within hours parents began calling physicians, newspapers, schools, and hospitals to find out where they could get the "anti-polio vaccine," as they called it. The mayor of New York City requested that President Eisenhower set up a system of federal supervision for allocation of the vaccine. And Eisenhower asked the State Department to transmit to the seventy-five countries with which the United States had diplomatic relations the details of producing the Salk vaccine. He also wanted to know how many of the precious doses were available to be sent abroad.

It was understood by the medical world, though not dictated, that children from age five to eight and pregnant women were at greatest risk and should be first in line for available doses. Exceptions, however, were numerous. Cutter Laboratories announced a special program to provide polio vaccine to all its workers and stockholders. Doctors reserved supplies for their own families and friends. That spring, a New York mother and her children were visiting her father in St. Louis. She wanted polio protection for her youngsters and knew she would never get the shots in New York, where the vaccine was scarce and where she had not lived long enough to establish a relationship with a pediatrician. She asked her father, a physician and research scientist, to call in his professional favors, and he did. A physician friend inoculated both her children in St. Louis, and when they packed up for New York City, they carried with them the next two doses, wrapped in dry ice, to be given at prescribed times later. That mother suffered guilt. Her sense of social responsibility and her desire for fairness told her that what was right was to stand in line and not shove. But her sense of mother-responsibility was satisfied. She may have elbowed in ahead of other deserving souls, but then neither of her children got polio.

ON APRIL 27, 1955, just fifteen days after the Ann Arbor announcement, fifteen days during which some four-hundred thousand polio inoculations had been given, the joking, the euphoria, and the shoving to get in line stopped and the fears, bigger than ever, were back. The front-page headline in the *Seattle Times* in oversized type read: "WESTERN FIRM'S SALK VACCINE WITHDRAWN AS EIGHT INOCULATED CHILDREN GET POLIO." The *New York Times* front-page headline was more conservative: "ONE FIRM'S VACCINE BARRED; 6 POLIO CASES ARE STUDIED." It would take days, then weeks, then years to sort out the facts, to place blame, to settle the lawsuits. Nonetheless, what seemed unthinkable that April proved true: children who had been vaccinated had come down with polio—six in California, two in Idaho. Before it was over, 204 so-called vaccine-associated cases occurred, about three-fourths of which were paralytic. Eleven people died. Most of the victims were in California and Idaho.

One of the Idaho children was eight-year-old Dorothy Crowley. She had been inoculated April 21 with the Cutter vaccine, along with almost four-hundred Clearwater County first- and second-graders. Within the week, she crawled onto her mother's lap and said, "I think I'm coming down with a cold. I ache all over." When her father, James Crowley, called the doctor, he said: "See if Dorothy can sit up without toppling. Then ask her to place her chin on her chest." When James went back to the telephone to report that Dorothy could do neither, the doctor ordered her to the hospital in Lewiston, fifty miles away. As her condition worsened and she went into an iron lung, news of more inoculated children coming down with polio reached her parents. One child died, then another. Dorothy spent two months in an iron lung and then was flown by MATS to the

Northwest Respirator Center on August 6, 1955. The pilot banked the plane to show her the mountains and the city, and she talked about that for days. In a couple of weeks Marcelle Dunning and Fred Plum and the rest of the staff had her out of the tank and onto a rocking bed. But she was still paralyzed, and they could work no miracle. Before long Dorothy was counted among the fatalities in what came to be called the Cutter "incident."

That some live virus might remain in batches of killed-virus vaccine had always been a possibility known to virologists, which was why extensive testing was done on each batch of vaccine for the field trial. The problem came with mass production and distribution of the vaccine. Laboratories, including Cutter, that had not participated in the field trial were among those making the vaccine for mass inoculations, and new ways to produce and kill the virus were being used that had not been tested outside of Salk's lab, where the batches were small and rarely left to stand for any length of time. As far as anyone knew, however, all the labs were using the same procedures. What, precisely, was the cause of the faulty Cutter vaccine, is not known. As Jane S. Smith wrote in her analysis of the event: "The responses to the Cutter incident . . . were predictable and unedifying. Without exception, everybody blamed somebody else." The NFIP, the government, Cutter, the AMA, and Salk all pointed fingers away from themselves.

Months of wrangling over new production standards for the vaccine and new inspection procedures followed. In the meantime, the vaccinations went on. Parents who had called their physicians at the first news of the bad Cutter vaccine were offered assurances of all sorts. Some of them were inaccurate, as was an account in Boulder's *Daily Camera* on April 28, the day after the news broke, which said that most likely those children had contracted the disease before the inoculations were given. Other people concluded, rightly or wrongly, that the problems were limited to vaccine coming from Cutter. In one way or another, enough parents were calmed so that by May 7, four million doses of poliomyelitis vaccine manufactured by five commercial laboratories had been administered, and without further incident.

Along with first- and second-graders all over the country, my brother lined up at Sacred Heart of Jesus that April to get his inoculation, administered by volunteer doctors and nurses rounded up by the county health department. The threat of a needle, the stranger giving the injection, the smell of alcohol—any of it might have made those schoolchildren anxious, but Kenny may have been among the most nervous. He was getting a shot for something his mother had and, though he tells me he wasn't sure what that meant, he was frightened. Being a kindergartner then, I don't remember getting the vaccine and may not have. If I did, it was not at school but in the office of a private physician. Boulder's doctors, however, like doctors everywhere else, were swamped with requests for the shots, but had only a small quantity. Karen McGinnis, whose mother came down with polio about the same time our mother did, can remember getting her Salk injection. She remembers the metal needle holder and the smell of alcohol. "I remember the anger and sense of unfairness and confusion and the questions," she told me. "Why now? Why couldn't the vaccine cure the effects of polio? Why not one year earlier? Why my mother? Why not me?"

With the vaccine approved and becoming more widely available, the unvaccinated continued to come down with polio. One woman's physician-husband brought home doses for his family, but held off administering them because of the Cutter tragedies. And then, with the vaccine in her refrigerator, the woman began to ache and her temperature rose and she knew it wasn't just the flu. Her bout with polio left her a quadriplegic, just like Bill Warwick, who was two days away from his scheduled vaccination when he came down with the disease in September 1955. Being an adult male, he was at the end of the line for inoculations.

By the close of 1955 polio began to decline. The vaccine brought a drastic drop—80 percent—in paralytic polio cases by 1957. By the fall of that year, 215 million doses of the vaccine had been released, and the 1957 polio rate was less than one-third what it had been in the previous six years. In a decade, the number of annual cases in the United States dropped from 38,000 to 570.

EFFORTS TO RAISE MONEY FOR POLIO RESEARCH and care of patients went on after the vaccine was approved, but it became an increasingly difficult battle. Celebrities still went on the air to appeal for dimes and dollars, and newspapers still made their annual January pitch. The tactics shifted, however. Now a newspaper story would run a photograph of a former polio patient and say something like: "If you've been thinking the Salk vaccine won the polio battle, and there's no need to wage war any longer, just talk to this woman who has needed $15,000 of March of Dimes funds since falling ill." The swimmer and actor Esther Williams urged television viewers to join the 1958 March of Dimes by saying that she, too, had "breathed a big sigh of gratitude" with the news of the Salk vaccine and thought "at last, polio is a thing of the past." But, she went on, "is polio a thing of the past for a paralyzed mother for whom the vaccine came too late? No." But the pleas were becoming strained. The public was tired of polio, and the NFIP knew it. On the same day that newspapers reported the successful vaccine, they ran a small story saying the NFIP would not go out of business, but would switch to some other field. Maybe mental health, Basil O'Connor was quoted as saying, but no decision had been made.

Not only was raising money for the polio cause increasingly difficult, but so was getting people vaccinated. The drive toward nationwide immunization never regained its momentum after the Cutter scare. The short supplies of 1955 turned into a surplus in 1957, and the NFIP had to work to lure citizens to take the vaccine they had waited so long for. That year, sixty-seven million people were in the top-priority bracket for the vaccine—people under 20 and pregnant women—but just twenty-five million had received the recommended three injections. In the fall of 1957 the *Journal of the American Medical Association* ran an editorial urging doctors to nudge patients to get their vaccines. Colored "reminder" cards were supplied free to all doctors as part of an "operation cleanup" organized by the AMA. Orange cards went to people under forty who had not been inoculated or had not completed the three-shot series. Thirty-seven million Americans still had not been vaccinated at all, and another forty-four million needed second or third injections.

Meanwhile, communities used a variety of methods to encourage vaccination. In Tennessee, schools that had closed for the summer reopened to serve as free vaccine clinics. In New York City, a district club of Democrats mailed postcards urging people to bring their friends and get a ninety-five-cent polio shot during the evening hours set up for adults. In Birmingham, Alabama, the county NFIP chapter threw a "vaccination before vacation party" to induce youngsters to get their inoculations, and thousands of children showed up at Kiddieland Park, where they were given free vaccines and then a pink slip that allowed them to climb on a ride for just five cents. Individuals, both celebrated and private, did what they could to entice Americans to make use of the vaccine they had so long anticipated. Elvis Presley agreed to be vaccinated in public to inspire his teenage fans to submit to the needle. HEW Secretary Marion B. Folsom warned: "If people will use the vaccine available, it is possible to give paralytic polio a knockout blow within the next year. It will be a tragedy if, simply because of public apathy, vaccine which might prevent paralysis or even death lies on the shelf unused." In Grand Rapids, Michigan, Frances Downing Vaughan wrote a letter to her local newspaper in 1957 urging young people to get their shots. She wrote, "I am compelled to add my personal plea to the current campaign for all young adults to receive the Salk vaccine. My only brother died of polio on my birthday last May [May 22, 1956, her thirty-fourth], leaving four little children. It was ironic that as a newspaperman he was well aware of the disease and heralded its ultimate conquest—and that he should die totally paralyzed and speechless from it. The vaccine was not available in time for him less than a year ago."

By the spring of 1958, as the polio season approached, at least 40 percent of preschool children had no protection against polio, and another 10 percent had fewer than the three doses. In August that year $25 million worth of vaccine was backlogged and in danger of passing its six-month expiration date. Although the polio rate had dropped to fifty-eight hundred in 1958, some physicians worried that the incidence of polio would rise because so many Americans had failed to get vaccinated.

In 1958 that seemed to be the case in Detroit, where a health emergency was declared to combat the city's worst outbreak of polio since 1955. Almost five hundred cases of polio, including fourteen deaths, drew attention to the fact that eight-hundred thousand of the area's three million people "had not bothered," as *Newsweek* put it that fall, "despite the U.S. Public Health Service's recent entreaties to the American public, to get even a single shot of Salk protection." The NFIP rushed doses of the vaccine to the city, where forty-five clinics offered the shots for one dollar for adults and fifty cents for children.

IN THE MEANTIME, the nation was getting its second polio protector in the form of a live, attenuated vaccine. In 1953, Albert B. Sabin reported to the NFIP's Immunization Committee his success with modifying virus virulence with the use of monkey kidney tissue, but by then the NFIP had already made plans to go ahead with the Salk field trial. Sabin was convinced that the live-virus vaccine ultimately would be the most effective method, but with the NFIP diverted elsewhere, he turned to the World Health Organization, which took up the task of pursuing the attenuated vaccine. Sabin reported in 1957 to the Fourth International Poliomyelitis Congress in Geneva that the live polio virus vaccine, administered by mouth, was potentially more effective in wiping out polio than the Salk vaccine. The Sabin vaccine had several advantages over the Salk one, principally that it was taken orally, which made it easier and quicker to administer and thus better suited to controlling epidemics. It also apparently produced greater and more lasting immunity without booster shots, and it had a further advantage in that the weakened live virus was shed in the feces of those vaccinated and spread immunization to others in the community. That aspect of the Sabin vaccine made it especially effective in areas where the disease was still endemic, mainly in underdeveloped countries. The refusal of the NFIP to back the live virus was seen by some as evidence of indifference toward the rest of the world. It seemed to say, polio is conquered in the United States, so why should we support a measure that might be more effective in controlling polio elsewhere?

By the early sixties the live vaccine was licensed by the United States Public Health Service, one strain at a time, but without fanfare. The decision had taken so long and polio had so retreated from public concern that it was all anticlimactic. By 1962 the Sabin vaccine replaced Salk's, both in the United States and abroad, as the preferred type. The baby boom generation lined up for their Sabin sugar cubes and hardly noticed that the Salk vaccine was disappearing.

While Salk's contribution had been to show that it was possible to achieve lasting immunity to a disease without acquiring it, the Sabin virus used long-held principles of immunology by causing an infection with a harmless strain of the virus and thus creating immunity to more dangerous strains. The ongoing problem with the live-virus vaccine, however, is that it carries a small but predictable risk of paralytic polio. One in four million doses contains a virus that has reverted to its contagious and paralytic state. Shed in the feces, just as the attenuated strains are, the virus can infect not only the person it was administered to but other susceptible people near the recipient. When the Sabin-type vaccine became the choice in the United States, the risk associated with it was known, but was considered insufficient reason to curtail its use. The recommendation from the advisory committee to the surgeon general for this change to the Sabin type also included a change in emphasis. Intensive immunization of infants and preschool children, the largest and most at-risk group, was to be the public health focus, not the oral vaccination of adults.

Experts have gone on to debate the relative contributions of Salk and Sabin, which was much discussed in the fifties and into the early sixties. Salk was criticized, called "too glib," a "fast-talker," an "opportunist." Sweet as the victory over polio was, one medical historian wrote:

> It left a slightly bitter taste in many mouths. The obvious scrambling of several participants to be the first to win the race and the intemperate attacks by some who took up the cudgels on behalf of one or another of the chief actors smacked of the arena rather than the scientific laboratory. Perhaps this is the American way to success; if so, one can only hope that we will eventually learn to concentrate more on conquering nature than on outshining each other.

Salk never received a Nobel Prize for his work, some say because his work was derivative rather than original. He also was never inducted into the National Academy of Sciences, though many other polio scientists were.

The debate over which of the vaccines—the live or the killed—is the most effective goes on even today. It is a controversy over the issues of risk versus efficacy. Although the Sabin type does include a risk of inflicting paralytic polio, it also provides a more lasting immunity. The debate arises because of the way the polio virus moves in the body and the different ways the two types of vaccines combat it. The polio virus first invades the intestines, where it lives, replicates, and usually establishes harmless infection. Sometimes, however, it moves from there to the bloodstream and thus finds the nervous system, where it does damage. The killed vaccine, Salk's, enters the bloodstream and raises antibodies that can then head off a virus before it reaches the nervous system. But because it never enters the intestines, it does not provide what doctors call "gut immunity," the raising of antibodies in the intestinal tissue. That means someone inoculated with the killed vaccine can still carry the virus in the intestines and pass it through feces to someone who is not inoculated.

The live vaccine, however, which is taken orally and goes directly to the intestines, does provide that gut immunity. In that way it not only prevents the vaccinated person from becoming a carrier of polio but also allows some of the vaccine virus to be excreted and immunize someone else. The picture is not complete, however, without knowing that if the virus mutates, which it sometimes does, the vaccine shed can cause the disease.

When it came time to vaccinate our children against polio, my husband and I couldn't face the live vaccine, which is the one pediatricians routinely dispense. No matter how small the risk, one in a few million even, it was too high for us. Jens and I had lost twice already at the polio roulette wheel, and we weren't going to take any chances with our sons. We had them twice inoculated with the inactivated poliovirus to help them build antibodies to the virus, and then followed up with the oral live vaccine, for the longer immunity.

THE NFIP's ROLE IN THE DEFEAT OF POLIO has been debated in medical circles for years. The historian John Paul concluded that the NFIP came on the scene "at a time when omens were favorable and the tide was running with ever-increasing strength in its favor. . . . It would be more than naive to maintain that the brilliant discoveries made between 1938 and 1953 that furthered the cause of vaccines for poliomyelitis were made as a direct result of the foundation's financial support—as some have so vociferously claimed." The public view was simpler: Salk, with March of Dimes money, brought an end to polio, and now we don't need to think of it again. Those grateful to have survived unscathed, as well as those with torturous memories and scars, seen and unseen, were eager to leave behind their memories of risk, fear, and loss. Hundreds of iron lungs, those emblems of the worst of the disease, were airlifted by MATS to distant countries where epidemics still flared; others gathered dust in hospital basements.

And if the public was no longer interested in the disease, then the NFIP couldn't be either. Marcelle Dunning in Seattle told me she had expected the disease to taper off after the Salk vaccine became available, but instead its ending was abrupt. Funding for the Northwest Respirator Center dried up in 1958, and the short-lived rehabilitation unit dissolved, along with others around the country. Wrote Jane S. Smith:

> Somehow, polio had ceased to be a vital concern. . . .
> Now it seemed that the public expected the past
> victims of polio to rise up and walk away, cured by a
> miracle of federal licensing. Once lionized as heroic
> examples of human fortitude, the thousands of polio
> survivors who continued to need medical and financial
> help were suddenly ignored as embarrassing emblems
> of their own poor timing, clumsy enough to get polio
> before the vaccine that could have protected them was
> found. As veterans of other wars would continue to
> discover, the same civilians who pray for them in the
> heat of battle don't like to be reminded of the wounded
> and the dead after the war is over.

As the drama to end polio was played out and concluded, as the nation turned its attention to new interests, my mother lay on her rocking bed, a witness only to what she could see from her window and into our kitchen and living room. She lay motionless and without hope of recovery.

CHAPTER NINE

Silences

There's a scene from my childhood in the Swedish film *My Life as a Dog*. It's an episode I'd forgotten until I went to see the movie in 1988, knowing it was about a boy whose mother dies and expecting it to stir in me the feelings I finally wanted stirred about mother loss. I lived in San Francisco then, alone for the first time in my life. My marriage of seventeen years was over except for the paperwork, and I had begun, finally, to review my past. All roads, I found, were leading to my mother, and I was beginning to mourn her loss.

As I watched the movie, knowing the boy who wanted to please his young mother was going to lose her, I reached for a tissue. And then came the brief scene that made me sit up straight and brought my mother's death day back to me. The boy had gone shopping for a gift for his ill mother—a toaster—and hurried home to deliver it, but before he could push open the door, a man, a family friend, opened it. It was the expression on his face, the man at the door with the face that said, "Your mother is dead," that I'd seen before. In my case, the man was my father.

It was April, an afternoon in 1956, and Kenny and I had been at school as usual. How we got home that day, or any other day, I don't know, but there I was at our back door, standing on the step, looking up at my father and knowing my mother was dead.

My father refused to let me and Kenny in. I can still see his face, pale and tensed, his eyes sad beyond weeping. He shooed us with his hand and we ran away. I don't know whether he actually said anything. Kenny ran up the alley to the Mileses', with Danny and Stevie chasing him.

I'd forgotten about Daddy at the back door until seeing *My Life as a Dog,* but two other memories of that day had stayed with me. One was being inside the back door of my grandparents' house in the midst of a group of adults. I must have gone there when Kenny ran away. I remember standing next to my grandmother, crying, and she was crying. I heard the doctor tell her he had a pill that would help her feel better. I remember feeling invisible, certainly unnoticed, in that circle of adults above me. I wailed inside my head, but not aloud: "Doesn't anybody know she's my *mother?*" I couldn't understand why the doctor was paying so much attention to my grandmother, why he didn't give *me* a pill, why no one seemed to know I was even there.

Another memory I've held through the years was being in Nita's arms, as she carried me to Mother's bedside. Our house was silent, with no one there but Nita, Mother, and me. Nita stood at the side of the rocking bed and held me in her arms. I looked down at Mother's face and closed eyes. She could have been asleep. In death she was hardly more still than she had been in life. Nita talked quietly, telling me Mother had died, telling me she would soon be taken away and I should say goodbye. I didn't understand. Whatever terrors I had imagined, from my father's face and grandmother's tears, apparently hadn't come to pass. Mother was there. She looked the same. Only the silence was different. "Why can't we just keep her?" I whispered to Nita. I didn't understand why someone would take her away or where she would go. Nita held me tight, murmuring in my ear. She allowed me one last look, one last private moment to say goodbye, even though I didn't understand why I had to.

Those are the memories I have of my mother's death day and all I knew of it for the next thirty-five years. Not how or why or when, exactly, she'd died.

NOT UNTIL I WAS IN MY LATE THIRTIES did I begin to ask the questions that would fill in the details. When I asked, in the summer of 1987, one of the first stories my grandmother told me was that a few days before Mother died she'd had a dream, a nightmare of being lost, of falling through darkness, and she'd called out in her dream to

Maurine. She kept calling "Mother, Mother," pleading for help from the descent. "But you didn't come," she had said to her mother, and the nightmare went on. When Maurine told me this, I heard regret in her voice and saw it in her eyes, focused somewhere past me. She was still taunted by the memory, as if she had in fact, not in a dream, failed to rescue her daughter.

Maurine tells me that the night before Mother died, Dad had not come home and so she slept on the couch in our living room, positioned, as always, so that all she had to do to see Mother was open an eye. When she awoke that morning, she saw Kenny asleep, again, on the rocking bed with Mother. This time when Maurine asked him why he had gotten on the bed, knowing it was against the rules, he'd said only that he'd awakened in the night and thought Mommy was lonesome.

That early morning, with the sun rising in the east window behind her head and coloring the room, Mother told Maurine she was afraid she was passing another kidney stone because she was in such awful pain. She wasn't sure she could endure another, knowing exactly what lay ahead. "I'd rather die," she said.

I've tried to imagine Mother's last night, her 674th on her back, supine and unmoving like a soldier at attention. Pain, from which she'd never been free, had returned in force to stretch out with her on the rocking bed, and there was no hope of escaping it. I wonder whether she knew this time was different, whether there was anything in the dark of that night, in that pain, to tell her she was entering her last hours.

The morning of the day Mother's life ended, Kenny and I went to school as usual. Then someone, probably Maurine, summoned a doctor and notified Dad's office, asking them to find him. The doctor arrived, and Maurine and Hayes and Nita stood by, watching as Mother's pain deepened. Dad's office tracked him down in Denver. When he walked in to call on clients, someone said, "Are you Del Black? You're wanted at home right away." Word was that Mother was "in trouble." Dad tells me he drove as fast as he dared between Denver and Boulder and arrived before lunch. As he remembers it, "She was fading fast." Someone also called Aunt

Sarah at her home in Denver, who called Katherine at her job and said, "She's dying. We've got to get to Boulder."

Mother's last hours were, apparently, a reenactment of the nightmare, except this time her mother knew she needed help but still could do nothing to stop her daughter's descent. Mother kept asking what time it was. When Katherine heard that later, from Maurine, she interpreted it as meaning that Mother was waiting for her children to come home from school. But no one retrieved us. No one plucked us from our classroom seats to take us to her. We sat through our lessons and lunch and the afternoon not knowing our Mother was dying and waiting to see us one last time. No one came for us so we might have a final look at our Mother's sentient face, might hear a final word.

Dad remembers that at the moment Mother died only he, Nita, and Maurine were in the house. And as Mother slipped away, Dad recalls, Maurine frantically slapped her face and begged her not to go, trying to stop what she knew was happening. I don't know whether or when the doctor returned to pronounce her dead. I suppose that she who could not breathe would have gone on breathing after death until someone turned off the machine.

Katherine and Sarah arrived too late. When they pulled up in front of our house, they heard Maurine crying, rushed in, and then stood at the foot of Mother's bed. They wept and prayed. It was, Dad remembers, "a hell of a nightmare," finishing his memories of that last day with a peculiar detail. He said that when it was all over, he ran outside to find Hayes and shake his hand and tell him how sorry he was. I hadn't known till then that my grandfather couldn't bear to be with his daughter as she died.

Dad also said he told the doctor he was going to "get bombed" that night. Apparently, the doctor put his arm around Dad and asked him to hold off. But Dad didn't. By then he'd found drinking "to be a pretty good crutch," and he was in need of a crutch that night.

My grandmother says that later, when the mortuary had taken Mother's body away, she and I sat together in her living room, with me on her lap, and cried. Helen Duhon came, though she can't remember whether she knew my mother had died or had just stopped by as she so often did, and found a doctor trying to comfort Maurine. Friends continued to gather and sat around the kitchen table with Maurine and Hayes. "Maurine didn't want to accept your mother's death," Helen told me recently. "She thought she could still go over there and do something."

My parents' marriage ended just short of ten years.

ON FRIDAY EVENING there was a Catholic rosary said for Mother at Howe Mortuary, lead by Father Charles Forsyth. For the lengthy service, Mother's casket was open. She lay against orchid-colored satin in a casket called a half-couch, the kind with a dutch door that allows the top of the body to be exposed and the bottom to be concealed. She wore a dress that belonged to Katherine. In the days after her death, while preparations were being made for her funeral and burial, someone wondered about what clothing to bury Mother in, and Dad offered that she liked yellow. She didn't have a yellow dress, but Katherine did, and gave it to her.

Katherine tells me that that evening, while the rosary was said, Maurine instructed Kenny and me each to touch Mother in her casket and place in her hand notes we had written. I have no memory of that and I have no idea what I might have written to her, but Katherine saw us do it. I was calm, maybe because I'd already seen Mother's body, but Kenny became "unglued," Katherine told me, when he touched Mother. He ran from the room, with Katherine right behind, and when she caught up with him, he sobbed and said, "They stuffed her."

The funeral was Saturday morning, 9:00 A.M. Two black limousines from Howe Mortuary picked us up in front of my grandparents' house on College Avenue and drove us to Sacred Heart of Jesus. The cruciform church with a cathedral-like spire was built in 1908 of local sandstone and stood next to the school Kenny and I attended. We had often knelt at mass with our classmates before the ornate altar painted white and gold and populated with colored statues. I'd been baptized there, at the huge baptismal font.

I remember the funeral, but my recollection only confirms what a rogue memory is. In my memory of the service I see the brightly lit altar of the church, the casket, the backs of the gathered mourners, and the priest, but I view it all from a point high in the back of the church, eye-level with the huge, rose stained-glass window above the front doors. Already I had distanced myself from the sorrowful events and from the pain of the six-year-old girl sitting in the front of the church.

Mother's casket was draped with a blanket of roses. Spelled out in flowers was the word *Mother*, a touch, Dad told me recently, he would not have chosen and found maudlin, but then he had had no part in arranging or paying for the funeral. I don't know whether Dad stuck around long enough in the following weeks to see the headstone go up, but I think it, too, would have annoyed him. Its most prominent feature is the word, in large block letters, *MOTHER*, flanked by two flowers, apparently representing Kenny and me.

She died between Easter and Mother's Day and was buried on an April morning under a pine tree in Green Mountain Cemetery in a grave blessed by a priest. Those who gathered at the cemetery prayed that her soul "and the souls of all the faithful departed, through the mercy of God, rest in peace." Her grave, a few blocks from the house she grew up in and the one she died in, is on the mesa that rises up to meet the mountains she loved. "You can heave your spirit into a mountain," the writer Annie Dillard has said, "and the mountain will keep it, folded, and not throw it back as some creeks will. The creeks are the world with all its stimulus and beauty; I live there. But the mountains are home." Mother did finally have a homecoming. She'd come home to Boulder and to its mountains, for good. And now I live in walking distance of the house she and I grew up in, the house she died in, her grave, and the mountains that enfold her spirit.

In my first conversation with Marcelle Dunning, on the telephone before visiting Seattle, she told me that discharging Mother had been a hard decision. There hadn't been enough research in the form of case studies to tell them what to expect, particularly in longevity, from a person as physically devastated as Mother who was cared for at home. It was a stunning idea to me that Mother might *not* have come home, that we might have missed those last months together. The thought raised new questions for me: If they had kept her in Seattle, would she have lived longer? Would it have mattered to her or to any of us? Again, I'm grateful to the team at the Northwest Respirator Center. They thought a mother was better off at home with her family, if at all possible and despite what might lie ahead, and I agree. Troubled as her last months on Tenth Street were, I, for one, wouldn't trade them for anything.

In that conversation Dunning also asked me what my mother died of, but it was a question I was hoping to ask her. Neither my grandmother nor my father could say, although Dad speculated that her heart gave out. I retrieved a copy of her death certificate from the Boulder County records expecting to find the answer there. In the blank for "immediate cause of death" was written "periplegia" [*sic*] due to "poliomyelitis, anterior." But when I related that to Dunning, she said, "She didn't die of polio. She survived polio." The form also noted that she'd had "gastritis" for the past twenty-four hours. A doctor's name was recorded on the certificate, someone who's a friend of my father-in-law and who still lives in Boulder. I called him, thinking he would surely be able to tell me about Mother's care and health in her last months, but he didn't remember her at all. And how, he said to me, could he ever forget a fully paralyzed polio patient? He guessed that maybe one of the other doctors in his practice had cared for her, but a check of his thorough medical records revealed not a hint of her as a patient. He could tell me nothing about Mother, and how his name came to be on her death certificate remains a mystery.

From the two clues I could give Dunning, Mother's pain on her death day and the mention of gastritis on her death certificate, she surmised that Mother had a mild bronchial pneumonia and a stress ulcer or other gastrointestinal bleeding. Dunning had seen other severely paralyzed people go in a similar quiet and unexpected way. Jack Clements told me that his wife also died suddenly. "Suddenly," he told me, "in the sense that it never occurred to me that she wouldn't just go right on living." He was out of town on business when he got the call. "I was stunned with disbelief," he told me. "There was no particular medical diagnosis. Unofficially it was a matter of fatigue at the long arduous battle. Up to that time . . . she had no health problems. She often said her only side effect was 'flat hair.' "

Mother's death certificate did, however, contain two disconcerting pieces of new information for me. Her death date is recorded as April 25 instead of April 24, which is on her gravestone. And although I'd always known that Virginia was her middle name and that she and I shared a first name, I thought her name was spelled *Katherine*, just like my maternal grandmother, great-grandmother, and great-great-grandmother. Her gravestone gives her name as only "K. Virginia Black." But on her death certificate is written "Kathryn." These two details seem fitting in an odd way. How sadly appropriate, given my family's silences, that I should go much of my life not knowing my mother's exact name and that I still don't know, for certain, her death date. Do I believe what is written in stone or recorded on an official document? Like so much else about her, there will be no knowing.

AFTER TALKING TO DUNNING about what medical complications might have caused Mother's death, I faced the question I really wanted answered, one that is more complicated and, ultimately, unanswerable. I wanted to know whether she gave up and brought on her own death. There was evidence to support that idea, once I went looking for it. Just as the notion once prevailed that polio patients could cure themselves with willpower, today we like to think that we have some control over death.

"Literally, she lost the will to live," Fred Plum, who had directed the Seattle center, told me when I called to ask what he remembered about my mother. "Although I don't know the biology of that," he added.

Not a single patient died at the Northwest Respirator Center, but about 10 percent died soon, within two years, after departure, including Mother. In an unpublished paper, Dunning wrote about that group and listed some of the physical problems they had, such as kidney stones, episodes of aspiration, and severe respiratory problems (such as pneumonia). Those patients, she wrote, didn't necessarily have different physical problems, however, from those "who succeeded," but rather seemed "to lack the initiative, drive, imagination and support systems to achieve what the more successful patients had."

In my research, I encountered many stories about polio patients who failed to carry on, who died early in their care without obvious medical complications. Those who related the stories used them as illustrations of people who had given up. There was the man, for example, who died just days after his wife asked for a divorce, and the woman in an iron lung who had made good progress but then died within a week of learning that her children would go into foster care because the relative who had been keeping them would do it no longer.

On the other side, most published accounts of polio survivors, as the historian Daniel Wilson found, are uplifting stories illustrating the life-saving positive attitudes of those who endured despite sometimes severe handicaps. Their determination, and that of many others I heard about, seemed to be a factor in their survival. One such patient was Al Jepson. He was thirty-four, married, the father of three children, and established in a career when polio left him as fully handicapped as my mother. He told of his first realization of his situation this way: "I was determined to concentrate my mind and body to do everything possible to regain my strength and recover to the fullest." His physical recovery was negligible, but his emotional triumph was such that he could write four decades later:

> All I can say is that I consider myself to be a very lucky
> man. I had wonderful parents, a good education in
> high school, an excellent college experience and edu-

cation, the job of my dreams with a top-notch firm, the love and support of a superb wife and family, the continuing support after I contracted polio of doctors, helpers, friends and co-workers, the most appreciated support of [my employer], and the good fortune through all of this to come out with an overall good philosophy of life.

He died at age seventy-five of a stroke.

I searched medical journals for something concrete to tell me whether individual will can, apart from suicide, affect the timing of one's death and found what's called the anniversary reaction. It's a phenomenon well accepted among sociologists, psychologists, doctors, and others who study death, in which illness and death become associated with symbolic occasions. Studies show, for instance, that a person may sicken or even die on reaching the age when a parent died. Other studies show that Jewish mortality dips 31 percent below normal before the religious holiday of Passover and peaks by the same amount afterward. Anyone who ministers to the dying, such as hospice or emergency care workers, can tell of a similar phenomenon in which people hang on to life past the point where it seems reasonable, waiting to die until, perhaps, a grandchild is born or a relative arrives from out of town.

Other evidence supports the idea that most of us possess a strong "will to live," whatever the odds or price. The physician Sherwin B. Nuland, the author of *How We Die*, contends that "we rarely go gentle into that good night." Even when someone yearns for a tranquil death, he says, "the basic instinct to stay alive is a far more powerful force." When I was in Seattle, Dunning took me to meet a polio survivor who, following her illness, lost her husband to mental illness and then her children to separate foster homes. In the decades since, she has suffered repeated life-threatening medical complications due to her paralysis, but fifty years later she persists, living on a respirator, attended by hired caregivers. "When it comes to the nitty-gritty, when it comes right down to it," she said, "you surprise yourself" with wanting to live despite it all. James Warwick told me that he once posed "that terrible question" to his brother, Bill: "Wouldn't you be better off dead?" The two were, he hastened to remind me, "very, very close brothers, buddies and friends." And what came from his brother was "a graceful, generous and sweet answer: 'Oh, no, life is very precious; I can still see, I can hear, speak, . . . admire two husky, healthy boys; nah, I'll take this over the alternative.' "

But even if death was a welcome release for my mother, I don't think that necessarily means she gave up, didn't love her family enough, lacked courage or strength of character. Who can draw the line between recognizing defeat and giving up? In their study of respirator patients at the Mary MacArthur Unit, researchers found that such conditions as kidney stones and cystitis often raised patients' anxieties about their survival, "and thus occasionally had a rather severe effect on the psychological condition of the patient. Further attacks of pain, reminiscent of the acute stage of illness, seemed more than patients could bear." Who can say what physical and psychic pain Mother had already endured or how much more she could endure? That other similarly handicapped people have lived decades beyond what she did doesn't mean she could have or should have. "If the suffering was severe or lasted long enough," wrote Eric Cassell, "it never leaves the memory." I have no doubt that Mother had endured unforgettable pain. Perhaps the prospect of fighting only to endure more *was* too much for her.

THE "MINUTE" MOTHER DIED, according to the head of the local March of Dimes chapter, Dad called and insisted all the NFIP's equipment be removed as quickly as possible from our house. He wanted nothing left. The mortuary came to remove Mother's body; the March of Dimes came to remove her breathing machines. And almost as quickly, Dad disappeared. What little family life we'd had in the small rental house on Tenth Street was dismantled abruptly. My grandparents and father had some discussions, I learned over the years, about what to do with Kenny and me. I've heard that my grandparents begged Dad to leave us with them, but I can't imagine he put up enough resistance to make begging necessary. Maurine told me that a friend of Mother's wanted to adopt me (apparently without my brother), but as Maurine said, "even your Dad wasn't in favor of that."

Whatever decisions or agreements were made, Kenny and I weren't told of them. Our bunk bed and belongings were moved across the backyard to Maurine and Hayes's house, and we were settled into a bedroom at the foot of their basement stairs. No one mentioned Dad to us or offered an explanation as to why and where he went. Although I would never have used the word *orphan* about Ken or myself, we were in deed, if not in fact, orphaned with our mother's death.

My memories of life with my mother are few, but the time after her death, even the first years, are much more clear and whole in my mind. With Kenny on the top bunk and me on the bottom, we resumed our lives. We ate dinner on TV trays in my grandparents' living room and watched *Friday Night Fights* and *The Hit Parade* on weekends. Sunday mornings Hayes read the newspaper, while Maurine, Kenny, and I went to mass. I organized my books and collection of ceramic animals on shelves in the basement. When the scent of chaos, triggered by reminders of loss and rejection, no matter how trivial, grew too strong, I went to the drawer in my grandmother's bureau where she kept her gloves and scarves. Although the drawer was already tidy, I'd dump the contents and start over. Sorting gloves, matching pairs, dividing cotton from leather, stacking them with the longest ones on the bottom. Then the scarves. I'd fold them precisely, placing them by size, color, and texture into the drawer. Breathing in the cologne and talc lingering on the scarves, imposing order where I could when my heart rattled with pandemonium.

Kenny and I went back to our classrooms at Sacred Heart, entering school each day between the Sacred Heart of Jesus statue and the mother-angel. Once I was sitting again at my wooden desk, Sister Marie said recently, she could hardly bear to look at me. She cried through the days following Mother's death, and the sight of me back in her classroom was wrenching for her. I suppose it's a reaction many people had to Kenny and me.

AFTER MOTHER'S DEATH, my grandparents, father, brother, and I spun free of each other, into separate orbits, unable to cope with our own grief, unable to help each other. We entered a realm of silence and lived there with the fact of Mother's death. We smelled it, feared it, walked around it daily, but never spoke of it. Mother—her life, her illness, her death—became the unnamed, the unknowable, as if she had never been. One of Maurine's friends told me that after Mother's death, if something was said about Virginia, my grandmother didn't respond. This friend also said it was years before she heard Maurine say her daughter's name again. Photographs and Mother's possessions—anything that might have prompted memories—vanished from my grandparents' home. Until recently the only photograph I'd seen of my mother after polio was the one in the newspaper clipping showing her return to Denver, kept in my great-aunt's diary. When I asked my grandmother for others recently, she conjured a despairing scene, telling me that soon after my mother's death, she gathered up all the pictures of her sick daughter, tore each one into tiny pieces, and threw them into the trash.

The silence deepened. I never heard the words "your mother" or "polio," which only contributed to the shame, the mystery, and the abandonment of Mother's death. As I was growing up, no one said to me, "Your mother would have loved that" or "You do that just like your mother," and certainly not "I miss her" or "I loved her" or "she loved you." We became people defined by loss, defined by what was not there rather than what was.

Obedient children, Kenny and I never asked about our mother, never talked of her between us, hardly ever even looked at the two photographs of the before-married her that continued to hang in Maurine and Hayes's house. I never spoke of her or heard of her, but in the first years, in the dark, alone, I allowed myself to miss her. I remember going to my bed in my grandparents' basement and placing a chair next to me for my guardian angel, as we were taught to do at school, but I hoped it would be Mother who would come in the night instead. I kept a silent vigil, hands out, waiting to be filled by her, begging God to return her to me, talking to her in my nightly prayers. I tried to imagine what heaven was like and what she might be doing. I considered long and hard what powers angels had, as I was convinced she was now an angel. Did she have the power to come back and visit me, to sit on that chair next to me? And if so, why *didn't* she? Or maybe she did, but only while I slept. I made bargains with

God, promising anything in exchange for her. And at every opportunity for wishing—blowing out birthday candles, breaking wishbones, and dropping coins in wishing wells—I asked for her.

In the years just after Mother's death, strong images blended with dreams. Throughout the second grade and into the third I was troubled by a recurrent nightmare. In it I stood in the cafeteria line at Sacred Heart with the other children, forming a wide line through the cavernous central hallway of the school's lower level. The line wound up three steps and bent to the left, into the cafeteria. Straight ahead was the girls' bathroom. In the dream I had on the school uniform, but beneath it I was naked and terrified someone would discover my disgrace. There in my grandparents' dark basement, I'd awaken from the dream, my throat thick with fear, and I'd make sure to put on underwear before pulling the uniform over it and going off to school.

Over the weeks, then months, then years, with both our parents gone, Kenny and I fashioned a facade. We even called our grandparents "Mom" and "Hayes," further confusing for others and for ourselves the issue of whom we lived with. Now and then the facade would crack. My grandfather sometimes mistakenly called me "Virginia," and I would freeze, looking at him, hopeful, wondering what had made him say her name. I'd wait, wanting him to say something about her, to speak her name again, but he'd hurry on, and I'd be aware more than ever of the empty place inside me. With Mother's death, we lost her, our father, and, in a way, our grandparents, too. They couldn't be "grand" to us, indulgent and playful. Instead, in the wake of their great loss, they became our disciplinarians, saddled with child rearing again.

Externally, however, my life appeared normal enough, and I became so accustomed to never speaking of Mother that I lost sight of the oddness of being reared by grandparents and rarely tried to explain my situation to anyone. And so I became an adult who had no name for her mother.

WHEN I BEGAN TO LOOK into my past, I thought my family's enduring method of coping with sorrow by shoving it aside was unusual, but I came to see it wasn't. It was the expected, socially sanctioned path, one that rests on a belief that what we can't see and don't speak of can't hurt us. I found, however, that what I couldn't see and didn't know about my past was dictating and diminishing my daily life. My family had unwittingly colluded with the rest of the world in an inadvertent and peculiar way to keep me from making sense of the events in our family and from healing my sorrow. A disease so virulent that it killed my mother and destroyed our family and killed or crippled thousands of others became incidental to the nation, erased from social consciousness once a vaccine was found. The silence in my family reflected the attitudes and practices of a society that praised people like us for behaving as if nothing were wrong, that valued stoicism and expected adults to protect children from feeling or witnessing emotion.

Several years ago, after my first long talk with my grandmother about our family history, I wrote at length in my journal. I noted dates and details I'd never heard or known before, and at the end of that entry wrote: "How can it be that she died?" It was then thirty-one years after her death.

Since then, I've talked to many people about their experiences with polio. Among those who left a powerful impression were Harriet and Gerry Stephens, who live in Boulder. Harriet contracted polio in October 1954, when their twin daughters were not yet two and their third daughter was six months old. Harriet was left with no useful muscle strength below her neck, except for part of her diaphragm, which allowed her to breathe as much as two or three hours without help. Their children are long-since grown, and Harriet and Gerry still live in the house they bought when Harriet came home from rehabilitation.

When I visited them, they showed me an old family album. I paged through the thick scrapbook that begins in the spring of 1948 with their engagement to be married. The album records the milestones of a family's life, a family like others in the fifties, with photos of the young couple, then baby pictures of twin girls and later a third daughter, newspaper clippings, greeting cards, photos of family gatherings. Then in November 1954 the photos show Harriet in an iron lung. The twins stand on vinyl-covered chairs to see and talk with their mother. And the album goes on recording both the ordinary events, such as birthdays and holidays, and the extraordinary, such as Harriet's airplane flight in a portable iron lung. Page after page, year after year, the album reveals family life. Always Gerry and Harriet are there, she in a wheelchair, a scarf concealing her tracheotomy hole, both smiling with their children, parents, other family members, and friends.

What struck me was that the album went on and on. An event so cataclysmic as Harriet's paralysis didn't stop their family life. I pored through the album with envy and admiration for the loyalty and tenacity evident. I kept it months beyond the week I'd asked to have it. Again and again I leafed through the Stephenses' lives. Harriet could no longer hold a camera to snap a photo or use scissors to clip from a newspaper, but she drove the keeping of the album, instructing others what to do and insisting it be done, even when she was first in the hospital and then in a rehabilitation center.

And Gerry, though glimmers of fatigue came through some snapshots of him, was there through it all, and still is. Polio, even at its most rapacious, was not powerful enough to do in the Stephens family, and they have the album of their history to prove it. This is, of course, the album I wish our family had kept. They are the family I wish we could have been.

The French writer Albert Camus once said: "What's true of all the evils in the world is true of plague as well. It helps men to rise above themselves." That is true of some men, but my father cannot be counted among them. Adversity brought out the worst in him. I believe him when he tells me he was his own worst enemy, that he was "young, stupid, and selfish." I believe him when he says no one could judge him more harshly than he has judged himself. And I can see that fate did, indeed, torment him. Nonetheless, what I wanted from him—and still want—was for him to have the heart and strength to stand up to his trials. Always, I've wanted more from him than he could or would give.

I find a measure of comfort in understanding that a crucial, missing element for my father was that he didn't know how much he was loved and needed by Mother, Kenny, and me. He thought that what he did didn't matter. He thought he was expendable, and he wasn't. He didn't know that we children needed a mother and a father, and that we had lost them both. And that it would always matter.

Visiting with the Stephenses also made me know, in a way I had not before, how much I wish my mother had lived even in her crippled condition. As a child wishing on stars or later bargaining with God for my mother's return, I always had her coming back to me as she was *before* polio. The option that she might have gone on living years or decades longer, even to this day, on her rocking bed had not occurred to me until I began to talk to other survivors and their families. Hearing about Al Jepson, Hank Steputis, Bill Warwick, and others who lived long helped me understand how much their lives meant to their families. But it was looking into Harriet Stephens's face and seeing for myself how alive and present she is despite her immobility that stirred that ancient ache and renewed the profound wish that my mother had had more of life, whatever her condition. I make that wish for both of us.

In his memoir, *In Love with Daylight*, the novelist Wilfrid Sheed, who lost the use of "one and two-thirds legs" to polio when he was a teenager, emerged from his illness having discovered "the master truth": "God, or the Great Whoever, has been so lavish in His gifts that you can lose some absolutely priceless ones, the equivalent of whole kingdoms, and still be indecently rich." He's right, of course, but for years, decades, I couldn't see beyond the loss of the priceless gift of my mother to the treasures I had. And only now that I have the blatant fortune of my husband and sons and the family life we share do I feel indecently rich. I often wonder whether the twenty-two months Mother lived with her many losses was enough time for her to turn away from lost kingdoms to see what remained for her. And I'm afraid not.

MY JOURNEY BACK has showed me that what I had suspected all my growing-up years was true: the silences of my father and grandparents compounded the loss of our mother for my brother and me. Ultimately and imperfectly, that discovery helped me begin to stop blaming them and to feel compassion for the losses they, too, suffered. The more I learned about my family's history and its context of polio, I began to see them in a new light. I began to realize that we each experienced our own pain beyond measure. I understood that it was pointless to try to decide whether the agony of a child who loses her mother is worse than the devastation of a mother who loses her child. Nor can the pain of a mother who is dying be measured against the suffering of a father who wishes to die and who loses himself and his family.

When I first heard that my grandmother had torn up the photographs that showed my mother in her iron lung or limp in her wheelchair, I was angry because I could see only that I had been denied a record of memories that I wanted. But now a mother myself, I can glimpse the mixture of anger and sorrow that must have driven her to destroy those painful reminders of her daughter's dying. I can only guess what despair she must have felt as she battled to preserve only the memories of her daughter as well and strong, with arms thrown wide to embrace us all.

My struggle now is to celebrate the happiness that is mine. I know, as only those to whom the worst has happened can know, that nothing lasts. Although I often fail, I nevertheless try to live each day grounded in a sense that these treasures, my husband and my sons above all, though fragile, are here now and mine to love.

CHAPTER   TEN

Aftermath

In the decades after the Salk vaccine was approved, polio became nothing more than a poignant oddity, one that eventually faded altogether from national consciousness. The disease was forgotten. It was not, however, gone. The vaccines, significant as they were, did not wipe out the disease nor its legacy. Some 250,000 people worldwide still contract polio each year, and a few countries still experience annual epidemics. As for the 1.4 million people living in the United States who survived polio, 25 percent have developed new problems stemming from the disease. And with time, more will. Polio is not gone for those thousands still contracting the disease around the world, nor for those thousands more who are living with old and new disabilities. Nor, of course, is polio gone for those of us, in numbers never counted, whose scars are unseen.

THE WORLD HAS SEEN A STEADY REDUCTION in polio since 1988, when the World Health Organization called for its global eradication by the year 2000. The United States has been free of the wild poliovirus since 1979. These days, all cases in the United States are the rare ones due to imported poliovirus or mutations in the live virus vaccine. The last known case in all the Americas was a Peruvian boy named Luis Fermin Tenorio who contracted polio in 1991. In the absence of any cases in the three years following, the Pan American Health Organization declared the region free of polio. In addition to the Americas, other areas reporting few or zero cases are Western Europe, countries of the Pacific and Pacific Rim, the Mahgreb countries of northern Africa, the Persian Gulf states, and many southern African countries. A high percentage of the world's cases come from a limited number of countries where the disease is endemic: India, Pakistan, Bangladesh, and Egypt.

Among world health authorities, the discussion is no longer whether the wild poliovirus can be eliminated, but when. The methods to stop it by the end of this century exist, but that may or may not happen, since eradication depends not only on the availability of resources but also on political will. The public health credo that "prevention is better and cheaper than cure" applies wholeheartedly to polio, a disease that can barely be treated and certainly not cured. Although smallpox is the only disease to have been eliminated from the world's natural environment, that success, led by the World Health Organization and culminating in 1977, raised expectations for the elimination of other diseases, chiefly polio. But polio is different from smallpox in several important ways that make its eradication more difficult. Smallpox, for example, has obvious, unmistakable symptoms; whereas most cases of polio have no significant symptoms, which means the disease goes undetected while spreading. A further complication is that several illnesses, including Guillain-Barré syndrome, cause poliolike paralysis. The only way to confirm a case of polio is by analyzing stool samples. To further complicate matters for health officials, the attenuated virus in the polio vaccine is nearly identical to the virus that causes paralysis, so health officials cannot test samples from the sewer to determine whether polio is present in an area. Virus in the feces of immunized people shows up in the analysis.

Differences in the smallpox and polio vaccines are significant also in the ease of elimination. The smallpox vaccine is heat stable—one dose lasts many years and leaves an obvious scar. The oral polio vaccine, however, is sensitive to heat, which makes it difficult to deliver effective doses in tropical and isolated areas, with multiple doses necessary for full protection.

In the 1950s, polio had the distinction of being the only serious epidemic disease in the Western world. And when its threat was eliminated, we acquired a kind of medical hubris that deepened with the subsequent elimination of smallpox. We began to think the threat of viral diseases had passed. Today, only a generation after the polio vaccine, AIDS has taught us humility. Not only have we failed to eliminate infectious diseases, but AIDS is worse than anything we've seen before. Sherwin Nuland, at Yale University, said flatly: "There has never been a disease as devastating as AIDS. My basis for making that statement is less the explosive nature of its appearance and global spread than the appalling pathophysiology of the pestilence. Medical science has never before confronted a microbe that destroys the very cells of the immune system whose job it is to coordinate the body's resistance to it."

The world will do well to free itself of polio as soon as possible. Not only will the humanitarian advantages be considerable, but so will the economic returns. The cost of treating even a fraction of those who need care is enough to pay for the total prevention of polio throughout the world. And by the turn of the century, we'll need all the resources we can muster—from the economic to the spiritual—because by then as many as 110 million people worldwide will have been infected with HIV.

IN THIS COUNTRY, and in all the others where the wild virus has been eliminated, we face a different polio problem. In the mid-1970s, and increasingly since then, adults who earlier in life had polio began turning up in their doctors' offices with vague but serious complaints: fatigue, exhaustion, muscle weakness, painful joints, difficulty breathing and sleeping, problems swallowing, and gastrointestinal difficulties. Along with such symptoms, for many, came fear, frustration, and anger because no one could say what was happening to them. Because polio had so long ago been dropped from everyday language and thought, even by doctors and even by some who had once had the disease, no one thought to link these new complaints to that old affliction. Many physicians treating today's patients have never seen an acute case of polio. Not until 1984 did the first International Symposium on the Late Effects of Poliomyelitis convene. There, the symptoms were recognized as an official syndrome and given a name: acute paralytic poliomyelitis sequelae, or postpolio syndrome. Even now, more than a decade later, the National Institutes of Health can define the syndrome only in vague terms: the development of new muscle weakness and fatigue in skeletal or bulbar-controlled muscles, unrelated to any other known cause, that begins between twenty-five and thirty years after an acute attack of paralytic polio.

Learning that polio, that long-ago disease they had battled and conquered, is behind these new problems that range from the inconvenient to the disabling, often brings on a new round of fear, frustration, and anger for people. The late effects are often reminiscent of the onset of the disease, not only in the physical symptoms but in the misdiagnoses, the frustration of not knowing what causes it or how to treat it or what the long-range prognosis might be.

This latest incarnation of polio is as varied as the original cases were. People whose conditions stabilized decades ago or who have lived all these years believing themselves fully recovered are stunned to find themselves relying on discarded crutches and braces or sitting in wheelchairs. One woman told me that until a couple of years ago no one would have known she once had polio, but now her legs are so weak she can no longer get into and out of the bathtub unassisted. With each passing year, she's able to do less.

Although nothing was said of it at the time, some scholars now think that Franklin Delano Roosevelt suffered postpolio syndrome. His polio-crippled body rapidly weakened at the end of his life, and he gave up even trying to suggest that he could stand. His hands, paralyzed at the onset of his disease, had quickly recovered nearly full strength and normal use. But by the end of 1944, months before his death, he could no longer hold a cup and saucer or light a cigarette himself. For some people left physically devastated by the disease, postpolio syndrome has come along to take away what little remaining useful movement they had. Harriet Stephens used her diaphragm to breathe on her own for two to four hours, which meant her family could take her out without coping with the respirator. Postpolio syndrome, however, put an end to that thirty years after her acute case of polio.

What causes the syndrome isn't clear, though it seems to be an accumulation of problems associated with years of impaired function.

Although one study showed some evidence of continued active disease in postpolio patients, few doctors believe there is persistent poliovirus infection or an immune problem. Some physicians dismiss postpolio problems as aging, though, of course, most people don't experience similarly debilitating symptoms until advanced ages, if at all. Some doctors have sent their patients to psychiatrists. Others have attributed the increased muscle weakness to overuse, suggesting, sometimes, that polio survivors are overachievers who have taxed their bodies beyond reasonable limits. "The very toughness on which the 'polios' prided themselves," wrote Jane S. Smith, "and on which they built their recovery, is now sending them back to the braces, wheelchairs, and respirators they struggled so energetically to discard."

Whatever postpolio syndrome is, it has everything to do with having had polio. The disease believed conquered decades ago has stepped forward for an encore. And, just as with the acute infection, it seems no one can do anything for the victims. Doctors suggest rest so that the sufferers will avoid overtiring already tired muscles. Anti-inflammatory drugs are sometimes prescribed to relieve pain; muscle-strengthening but nonfatiguing exercises are suggested. But that's about it.

What's also not clear is who among those not yet experiencing postpolio syndrome is likely to do so as the years go on. No one has studied the issue, but based on clinical observations it appears that those with the most severe residual paralysis are the most at risk, and the weakest limbs show the symptoms first. Patients with residual bulbar and respiratory weakness are at risk of bulbar and respiratory difficulties. And it appears that symptoms occur earlier in patients who had acute polio as older children than in patients who had the disease as infants.

We will never know the answers to many questions about polio—why, even, it was a summertime disease. The conversations and questions about polio stopped in midsentence. I kept turning up reports of interesting scientific studies in progress in the 1950s, most funded by the NFIP, that were discontinued after the vaccines were in use. No one can ever know what the completion of some of this research might have meant to today's polio survivors or to the treatment of postpolio syndrome.

A writer for *Time* magazine suggested recently that one positive side to postpolio syndrome is that it gives many patients an opportunity to come to terms with long-repressed emotions. Polio has been forgotten or pushed aside not only by the public but sometimes by sufferers themselves. Their new physical problems have sent them by the thousands into postpolio support groups, where they've not only discussed their new physical limitations but revisited their memories of being hospitalized for weeks, months, or years, of being at home watching from a window while the neighborhood children played ball. "Many of us never got a chance to mourn our losses," said one woman who has spent her life since polio in a wheelchair.

Mourning what's lost is something our society doesn't seem to value. Instead, we Americans place great stock in "getting on with it," an attitude FDR epitomized. Hugh Gallagher, the Roosevelt biographer who had polio himself, says the four-term president "shook his fist at the fates and seemed psychologically unable to acknowledge the permanence of his paralytic condition." Through tremendous effort, Gallagher contends, FDR convinced "his family, his party, the press, and the country that his paralysis was unimportant. Furthermore, he had convinced himself of this. . . . No matter how much he denied it—to himself and to the world—he was, indeed, a crippled man. The attack of polio that caused his condition was the central event of his life; his illness and lengthy rehabilitation shaped and altered his character." The official government position, however, was that polio was an episode in Roosevelt's life, one with no lasting effects. The public perception, certainly, was that FDR had overcome polio. But, as Gallagher noted, "A visible paralytic handicap affects every relationship, alters the attitudes of others, and challenges one's self-esteem. It requires meticulous minute-by-minute monitoring and control to an extent quite unperceived and unimaginable by the able-bodied."

When Roosevelt's Hyde Park, New York, home became a museum under the care of the National Park Service after his death, his leg braces, well worn and painted black at the ankles so as not to shine against his black socks, went on display, and then were removed. Museum curators decided, wrote Gallagher, "with exquisite sensibility that visitors might find this graphic evidence of the President's infirmity 'offensive.' " Even today, fifty years after his death, discussions about erecting a memorial to FDR include a debate over how to depict him physically—as the cripple he was or with his disability hidden, as it was in his public life.

Historians have viewed polio, if they've looked at it at all, in the same way—as an episode in American life. The period of the most severe epidemics, 1942 through 1953, and then the advent of the vaccines, were important wartime and postwar years, and those aspects of the period have overshadowed polio as a topic for historians. So thoroughly have we expunged polio from our memory that today the historian David Halberstam could write an eight-hundred-page social history of the fifties without addressing the disease, not even the discovery of the vaccines.

OVER THE YEARS OF COLLECTING CASE HISTORIES, anecdotes, and memories of others, as well as probing for my own, I've seen the varieties of losses individuals have suffered in the wake of the polio epidemics. Some lost movement of limbs and whole bodies, the capacity to breathe for themselves. Some lost the ability to do all but think, speak, blink, and feel pain. Some, like me, lost mothers or children, brothers, wives, husbands, friends. And in the aftermath of this disease, each of us has struggled to find the ways and means to live with our losses. Sharon Stern was one of scores of people who wrote to me in response to newspaper requests I made for memories of polio. She sent reminiscences spanning her forty years as a respiratory quadriplegic. In her letter, she asked what made me interested in polio. "Are you one of us?" she asked, meaning, I suppose, was I crippled from polio. Whatever she meant, my answer is, "Yes, I am."

All of us who lost something to polio have had to learn something about acceptance and about responding to challenge. In his study of polio narratives, the historian Daniel Wilson noted that despite the pattern of published stories ending on a note of reconciliation or affirmation, "if not triumph," polio's lasting legacy is the struggle it demands over the years. The struggle is to sustain the affirmation or triumph "over a lifetime marked by pain, disability, and limitation. . . . The surrender must be made again and again as the disability evolves." Just as those who lost the use of their limbs or lungs to polio have had to surrender repeatedly, so have those of us who lost loved ones.

I once spoke to my father about the what-ifs, the ultimate one being, "What if Mother had never had polio, had not died?" And he said something that had never occurred to me: "It might have been worse." I can't imagine how, and yet I've learned enough about the scope of suffering not to be so unwise as to long for some other than my own. What I know most certainly is that out of my mother's death has come the person I am now, with the life I have now, and I am grateful for both. The family Jens and I made grew out of the bond formed in our late mourning of our mothers' deaths. That I now live and am raising my children in a house situated between the one my mother died in and her grave is neither a coincidence nor incidental. It is, for me, a daily reminder that I embrace the past I hid from for so long and that from a sorrowful past a rich and gratifying future may be forged.

In the mid-1980s, thirty years after his mother's death and before he and I found one another again, Jens created a memorial for his mother of stone and wildflowers at the edge of a high mountain meadow near Boulder. Like me, he had lived thirty years unconsciously repressing memories of his mother and the sadness of her sudden death. She was cremated and has no grave, so he made a shrine to give himself a place to mourn her.

He took me to the memorial long ago, and it was there that I saw for the first time that my own mother's death was not a distant, irrelevant secret from my past but a constant presence that shadowed my days. In the years since then, Jens and I have taken our sons to that meadow in celebration of our gifts and in acknowledgment of our losses.

Jens's meadow memorial is a powerful symbol for me, a motherless child, and for the nation that lost so many to the disease that was forgotten. There is no grave for polio, no memorial for its dead, no quilt with the names of the polio veterans, no place where survivors can gather and mourn. There has been no national mourning. It falls to those of us who are wounded by the disease to raise our own memorials.

EPILOGUE

There is much I will never know about my mother. I began this book expecting that by the end of it I would have given substance to her outline, but I still feel more comfortable writing or saying "my mother" than "Mother." But something I have learned is that she has always been with me, and still is, in the love I hold for her. I will never know her, except as a child knows her mother, but I will always love her. My husband's father has kept the text of the eulogy from the 1954 funeral of his wife, Mary Ellen Husted. The minister at the First Congregational Church in Boulder said: "It is love that will keep . . . Mary Ellen alive in the hearts of all of us who knew her . . . It is not memory that keeps love alive, it is love itself which cannot die." I found this to be true for my mother as well. My love for her, I've found, is something distinct from my memories of her.

I wrote this book in an effort to create order out of the dissonance of my past, a past I could not accept, in part, because it was so unfamiliar. I wanted to create a history for myself, but also to give voice and face to all of us who suffered from polio, all of us who played our part, however unwillingly, in a significant period of American history. Franz Kafka said that a book should serve as "the ax for the frozen sea inside us." Writing this book has been my ax.

APPENDIX

For information about the late effects of polio, contact:

Gazette International Networking Institute/International Polio Network
4207 Lindell Blvd. #110
St. Louis, MO 63118-2915
314/534-0475
Provides written material about postpolio syndrome; keeps a national directory of support groups, health professionals, and clinics serving polio survivors; and publishes a newsletter called "Polio Network News," available by subscription.

———

Roosevelt Warm Springs Institute for Rehabilitation
P.O. Box 1000
Warm Springs, GA 31830
706/655-5300
Provides written information, conducts medical evaluations, and offers a clinic for those with postpolio syndrome.

———

The Polio Society
4200 Wisconsin Ave. NW, Suite 106273
Washington, DC 20016
301/897-8180
Provides medical and other information to the public and to health-care professionals, sponsors national conferences about postpolio issues, publishes a quarterly newsletter called "Options" (available with membership), and sponsors support group meetings in the Washington, D.C., area.

———

Lauro Halstead, M.D., M.P.H.
Director, Post–Polio Program
National Rehabilitation Hospital
102 Irving St. NW
Washington, DC 20010
202/877-1653

NOTES

Chapter One: Backache

p. 4 *The forties had brought* . . . : Barbara Lambesis, "Memorial Hospital History," *Arizona Medicine* (July 1976): 592–97.

p. 5 *in 1954 the city* . . . : *Arizona Republic*, 24 August 1954, 2.

p. 9 *When Mother fell ill* . . . : *Arizona Republic*, 12 June 1954, 8.

p. 10 *The hospital had begun as* . . . : Background on Phoenix Memorial Hospital came from an unpublished oral history by the former hospital administrator Mary Bennett, housed in the Arizona Collection, Department of Archives and Manuscripts, Arizona State University; an interview with George Scharf, a former pathologist at Phoenix Memorial Hospital; "Miracle on 7th Avenue: A History of Phoenix Memorial Hospital," *Today Magazine* (Fall 1981) n.p.; and Lambesis, "Memorial Hospital History."

p. 17 *Under normal circumstances* . . . : "Paralysis Patients Saved," *Science News Letter* 45 (1 January 1944): 2.

p. 17 *Iron lungs also posed risks* . . . : B. G. Ferris Jr., P. A. M. Auld, L. Cronkite, H. S. Kaufman, R. B. Kearsley, M. Prizer, and L. Weinstein, "Life Threatening Poliomyelitis," *The New England Journal of Medicine* 262 (25 February 1960): 371–80.

p. 18 *The overall mortality rate* . . . : Ibid.

Chapter Two: Epidemic of Fear

p. 20 *Trouble for the Hoovers started* . . . : Martha Hoover, interview with author, 8 November 1990.

p. 23 *Until the twentieth century* . . . : John R. Paul, *A History of Poliomyelitis* (New Haven, Conn.: Yale University Press, 1971), 2, 10–12. Alfred Jay Bollett, *Plagues and Poxes: The Rise and Fall of Epidemic Disease* (New York: Demos Publications, 1987), 151.

p. 23 *For centuries, other childhood afflictions* . . . : Paul, *History of Poliomyelitis*, 11.

p. 23 *An Egyptian stele* . . . : Ibid., 12.

p. 23 *Not until the end of the eighteenth* . . . : Ibid., 16.

p. 23 *not until 1887* . . . : Harry F. Dowling, *Fighting Infection: Conquests of the Twentieth Century* (Cambridge, Mass.: Harvard University Press, 1977), 204.

p. 24 *In August 1921* . . . : A detailed account of Franklin Roosevelt's polio experience can be found in Geoffrey C. Ward, *A First-Class Temperament: The Emergence of Franklin Roosevelt* (New York: Harper & Row, 1989). A summary can be found in Victor Cohn, *Four Billion Dimes* (Minneapolis: Minneapolis Star and Tribune, 1955).

p. 25 *On the evening of January 30, 1934* . . . : Ibid., 43–44.

p. 25 *With fanfare, the president* . . . : Dowling, *Fighting Infection*, 208.

p. 25 *The singer Eddie Cantor* . . . : Cohn, *Four Billion Dimes*, 52–53.

p. 26 *In January 1942* . . . : "Child Paralysis Rise Viewed as Alarming. Dr. Curran Hopes for 'Most Effective' Fund Drive This Year," *New York Times*, 6 January 1942, p. 16, col. 8.

p. 26 *In one week in August 1946* . . . : "The Polio Scourge," *Newsweek*, 19 August 1946, 23.

p. 26 *The disease crept into Tom Green County* . . . : Steven M. Spencer, "Where Are We Now on Polio?" *Saturday Evening Post*, 17 September 1949, 26.

p. 26 *As countries such as the United States* . . . .: Dowling, *Fighting Infection*, 209.

p. 27 *The Swedish epidemic* . . . : J. Nugent, "Stalking a Killer Virus," *The Rotarian*, April 1987, n.p.

p. 27 *In 1916, 95 percent* . . . : Paul, *History of Poliomyelitis*, 347.

p. 27 *By 1955, 25 percent* . . . : "Strange Facts about Polio," material provided for newspapers by the National Foundation for Infantile Paralysis. Appeared in the *Daily Camera*, Boulder, Colorado, 31 January 1956, n.p.

p. 27 *In 1953 in King County* . . . : *Seattle Times*, 17 January 1954.

p. 28 *The term* infantile paralysis . . . : Paul, *History of Poliomyelitis*, 346–47.

p. 28 *The disease came into its strength* . . . : Bureau of the Census *Statistical Abstract of the United States*, 1958 (Washington, D.C.: GPO, 1958), table no. 96.

p. 28 *In 1946 the Midwest* . . . : *Newsweek*, 19 August 1946, 22–23.

p. 28 *In a single week in 1946* . . . : Ibid.

p. 28 *Between 1948 and 1955* . . . : "Strange Facts about Polio."

p. 28 *In the summer of 1955* . . . : This fact from Ferris, "Life Threatening Polio-myelitis", p. 371; the rest of the material about the Boston epidemic of 1955 from Betty Levin (February 2, 1944, interview with author), William Tisdale (tape recording received December 1993), and Thomas J. Whitfield (January 29, 1994, interview with author).

p. 30 *Nineteen thousand people* . . . : *Statistical Abstracts*, 1951.

p. 30 *By midsummer of 1949* . . . : "Polio: Summer Season Brings Epidemics of This Uncontrollable Disease," *Life*, 15 August 1949, 47.

p. 30 *Mild cases went unreported* . . . : Paul, *History of Poliomyelitis*, 400.

p. 31 *Even during the worst epidemic years* . . . : "Simple Approach Is Urged by Dr. Leona Baumgartner at St. Louis Health Session," *New York Times*, 31 October 1950, p. 29, col. 6.

p. 31 *A child under ten* . . . : Howard A. Howe, "Are You Afraid of Polio?" *Harper's*, June 1945, 646–53.

p. 31 *The year my mother fell ill* . . . : Arizona State Health Department, interview with author.

p. 32 *"Even though this is estimated* . . . *"*: Paul, *History of Poliomyelitis, 4.*

p. 32 *Polio can circulate* . . . : F. C. Robbins, "Eradication of Polio in the Americas," *Journal of the American Medical Association* 270, no. 15 (20 October 1993): 1857–59.

p. 32 *Medical researchers have long thought* . . . : Paul, *History of Poliomyelitis, 2.*

p. 32 *In fact, considering the almost universal spread* . . . : Ibid.

p. 32 *After studying the 1944 Buffalo, New York,* . . . : "Maybe You Had Polio," *Newsweek*, 7 January 1946, 81–82.

p. 33 *The onset was bewildering* . . . : Betty Levin, interview with author, 2 February 1994.

p. 34 *Late one night during the summer* . . . : Thomas Whitfield, M.D., interview with author, 29 January 1994.

p. 34 *James and William Warwick received* . . . : James Warwick, letter to author, 20 January 1994.

p. 35 *Unaccountably, it affects* . . . : "Poliomyelitis," in *Mosby's Medical and Nursing Dictionary*, 2nd edition, The Health Reference Center, InfoTrac (St. Louis, Mo: C. V. Mosby Company, 1986), available from Information Access Company.

p. 35 *Betty Levin had been hospitalized* . . . : Levin, interview with author.

p. 35 *Mary Bready of Baltimore* . . . : Mary H. Bready, unpublished memoirs.

p. 36 *In 1949 one* Saturday Evening Post *writer noted* . . . : Steven M. Spencer, "Where Are We Now on Polio?" *Saturday Evening Post*, 17 September 1949, 27.

p. 36 *In the thirties some widely* . . . : Dowling, *Fighting Infection*, 205.

p. 36 *In 1936, the physician Charles Armstrong* . . . : Cohn, *Four Billion Dimes*, 4.

p. 37 *One epidemiologist studying* . . . : *Rocky Mountain News*, 11 August 1946, 25.

p. 37 *Then three laboratories, including the Yale* . . . : Paul, *History of Poliomyelitis*, 291–99.

p. 39 *Current understanding is that polio* . . . : Ibid., 2.

p. 39 *Researchers studying epidemics* . . . : "Maybe You Had Polio," 81–82.

p. 40 *Alex Coffin, who was born in 1936, remembers* . . . : Alex Coffin, letter to author, 2 February 1994.

p. 40 *The* Minneapolis Daily Times *ran a full page* . . . : "The Polio Scourge," *Newsweek*, 19 August 1946, 22–24.

p. 41 *As did many other summer camps* . . . : Charles A. Miller, *A Catawba Assembly* (New Market, Va.: Trackaday, 1973), 138–40.

p. 42 *When* Life *magazine listed polio* . . . : "Polio: Summer Season Brings Epidemics," 48.

p. 42 *Parents were told to teach their children* . . . : "Pain of Polio Relieved," *Science News Letter*, 2 September 1944, 146.

p. 43 *pregnancy and even daily routines* . . . : Spencer, "Where Are We Now?," 89.

p. 43 *One NFIP epidemiologist further speculated* . . . : *Rocky Mountain News*, 11 August 1946, 25.

p. 43 *The medical literature reported dramatic . . .* : Paul, *History of Poliomyelitis*, 187–89.

p. 43 *The physician for Frances Billings . . .* : Frances Billings Finke, letter to author, 16 June 1994.

p. 44 *In 1949, John A. Toomey . . .* : "Dr. Toomey Views Mystery of Polio," *Cleveland Plain Dealer*, 7 August 1949, n.p.

p. 45 *During the epidemic in Hickory, ...*: Robert Haywood Morrison, letter to author, 3 March 1994.

p. 45 *From the moment cases began to be listed . . .* : Patricia Lovett, letter to author, 17 December 1993.

p. 46 *A 1947 brochure directed at parents . . .* : "A Message to Parents about Infantile Paralysis," brochure, NFIP, 1947.

p. 46 *One magazine called polio . . .* : "Vitamin E Hailed as Possible Cure for Hopeless Disease," *Science News Letter*, 10 February 1940, 85.

p. 47 *In August 1949 . . .* : *Cleveland Plain Dealer*, 10 August 1949, 3.

p. 47 *Between 1947 and 1953 . . .* : Jane S. Smith, *Patenting the Sun: Polio and the Salk Vaccine* (New York: Morrow, 1990), 86.

p. 47 *Thinking of his paralyzed . . .* : Fred Davis, *Passage through Crisis: Polio Victims and Their Families* (Indianapolis: Bobbs-Merrill, 1963), 41.

p. 47 *Fred Davis, a sociologist . . .* : Ibid.

p. 48 *Parents of stricken children . . .* : Ibid., 36–37.

CHAPTER THREE: WAITING

p. 51 *In his memoir . . .* : Robert F. Hall, *Through the Storm: A Polio Story* (St. Cloud, Minn.: North Star Press, 1990).

p. 53 *Some children, like the nine-year-old . . .* : Sharon Stern, letter to author, 2 February 1994.

p. 53 *The father of Frances Billings Finke . . .* : Frances Billings Finke, letter to author, 16 June 1994.

p. 54 *Sid Moody, who came down . . .* : Sid Moody, letter to author, 30 March 1994.

p. 54 *At a Michigan hospital* . . . : Ruth Hazen, letter to author, 16 April 1994.

p. 54 *Like Mother, Louis Sternburg,* . . . : Louis Sternburg, Dorothy Sternburg, and Monica Dickens, *View from the Seesaw,* (New York: Dodd, Mead, 1986), 22.

p. 56 *Arnold Beisser, a recent graduate* . . . : Arnold R. Beisser, *Flying without Wings: Personal Reflections on Being Disabled* (New York: Doubleday, 1989), 23.

p. 57 *Fred Davis wrote of the shock* . . . : Fred Davis, *Passage through Crisis: Polio Victims and Their Families* (Indianapolis: Bobbs-Merrill, 1963), 17–19.

p. 60 *Arnold Beisser found that* . . . : Beisser, *Flying without Wings,* 5.

p. 60 *"The notions of personal* . . . *"*: Howard Brody, *Stories of Sickness* (New Haven, Conn.: Yale University Press, 1987), 92–93.

p. 60 *One young woman, a quadriplegic* . . . : "Young Mother, Polio Victim, Returns Home through March of Dimes Help," *Boulder Daily Camera,* 28 January 1954, 21.

p. 62 *In his book* The Nature of Suffering . . . : Eric J. Cassell, *The Nature of Suffering: And the Goals of Medicine* (New York: Oxford University Press, 1991), 34.

p. 63 *According to Cassell, people* . . . : Ibid., 36.

p. 63 *By July 1954, Arizona* . . . : "Five Polio Cases are Reported for Arizona," *Arizona Republic,* 2 July 1954, 10. Reports of additional patients are from subsequent issues of the *Arizona Republic,* specifically, 13 July 1954, 4; 17 July 1954, 1; 3 August 1954; 29 August 1954, 7; 3 September 1954, 10; 25 September 1954.

p. 64 *In late August, three months* . . . : "Phoenix Girl Dies of Polio," *Arizona Republic,* 8 September 1954, 1.

p. 64 *Thomas Karwaki was a* . . . : Thomas Karwaki, letter to author, 10 May 1994.

p. 64 *Ill in the epidemic of 1955* . . . : Sternburg, *View from the Seesaw,* 21.

p. 65 *When New Yorker Joseph Boettjer's young daughter* . . . : Joseph Boettjer, letter to author, 7 March 1994.

p. 66 *Karen McGinnis, whose mother* . . . : Karen McGinnis, letter to author, 4 October 1994.

p. 67 *Sharon Stern came down with polio* . . . : Sharon Stern, letter to author, 2 February 1994.

p. 67 *That separation caused pain* . . . : Thomas Whitfield, interview with author, 29 January 1994.

p. 67 *Doris Seligman, a teenager* . . . : Doris Seligman, letter to author, 7 May 1994.

p. 67 *For months, Ohioan Jack Clements* . . . : Jack Clements, letter to author, 9 June 1994.

p. 69 *Six-year-old David Heming* . . . : David Heming, letter to author, 7 February 1994.

p. 70 *Sharon Stern's mother came* . . . : Stern, letter to author.

p. 70 *Five thousand people* . . . : "World Bids Emilie Dionne Goodby," *Arizona Republic*, 8 August 1954, 1.

p. 71 *Fred Davis reported* . . . : Davis, *Passage through Crisis*, 176.

p. 71 *Arnold Beisser, rendered* . . . : Beisser, *Flying without Wings*, 167.

p. 71 *"At times I felt* . . . *"*: Ibid., 33.

p. 72 *To Beisser, only his head* . . . : Ibid., 19.

p. 72 *The iron respirators, those life-saving* . . . : This history of the tank respirator was drawn from John R. Paul, *A History of Poliomyelitis*, (New Haven, Conn.: Yale University Press, 1971), 325–31; Philip A. Drinker and Charles F. McKhann III, "The Iron Lung: First Practical Means of Respiratory Support," *Journal of the American Medical Association* 255 (21 March 1986): 1476–81; Philip Drinker and Charles F. McKhann, "The Use of a New Apparatus for the Prolonged Administration of Artificial Respiration: A Fatal Case of Poliomyelitis," *Journal of the American Medical Association* 92 (18 May 1929): 1658–60, reprinted in *JAMA* 255 (21 March 1986): 1473–75; and Catherine D. Bowen, *Family Portrait* (Boston: Little Brown, 1970), 237–43.

p. 74 *The Los Angeles County Hospital in 1948* . . . : Spencer, "Where Are We Now on Polio?," *Saturday Evening Post*, 17 September 1949, 90.

p. 74 *When an epidemic hit Massachusetts* . . . : "Strange Facts about Polio," National Foundation for Infantile Paralysis, in *Boulder Daily Camera*, 31 January 1956.

p. 74 *In Michigan's Upper Peninsula* . . . : Donald M. D. Thurber, letter to author, 14 January 1994.

p. 74 *At the 1933–34 Chicago World's Fair* . . . : Bowen, *Family Portrait*, 242–43.

p. 77 *In January 1953 the NFIP* . . . : Stanley Ulanoff, *MATS: The Story of the Military Air Transport Service* (New York: Franklin Watts, 1964), 113.

CHAPTER FOUR: HOT PACKS, EXERCISE, AND PRAYER

p. 80 *Taking note of those worse off* . . . : Fred Davis, *Passage through Crisis: Polio Victims and Their Families* (Indianapolis: Bobbs-Merrill, 1963), 137.

p. 80 *Patients at Warm Springs* . . . : Ken Purdy, " ' . . . the rest of me is alive,' " *McCall's*, October 1953, 60.

p. 81 *In 1950,* Collier's *magazine* . . . : Albert Q. Maisel, "If Polio Strikes Is Your Town Ready?" *Collier's*, 27 May 1950, 13–14, 70–72.

p. 82 *Frances Billings Finke, who fell ill* . . . : Frances Billings Finke, letter to author, 16 June 1994.

p. 83 *Another medical authority* . . . : Hugh Gregory Gallagher, *FDR's Splendid Deception* (New York: Dodd, Mead, 1985), 31.

p. 83 *"The best that could be said* . . . *"*: John R. Paul, *A History of Poliomyelitis* (New Haven, Conn.: Yale University Press, 1971), 324.

p. 84 *"In retrospect," wrote Paul* . . . : Ibid., 344.

p. 85 *Soon after her arrival* . . . : Robert D. Potter, "Sister Kenny's Treatment for Infantile Paralysis," *American Weekly*, 17 August 1941, 4.

p. 85 *Again and again the extraordinary nurse* . . . : Victor Cohn, *Sister Kenny: The Woman Who Challenged the Doctors* (Minneapolis: University of Minnesota Press, 1975), 178.

p. 85 *Scenes like one played out* . . . : Ibid., 175–76.

p. 86 *Still, many of her critics* . . . : Ibid., 145.

p. 86 *When* Sister Kenny *opened* . . . : Ibid., photo caption, n.p.

p. 86 *In fact, Carolee Cornelius Burris* . . . : Carolee Cornelius Burris, letter to author, 18 December 1993.

p. 87 *Writing in* Harper's *magazine* . . . : Howard A. Howe, "Are You Afraid of Polio?" *Harper's*, April 1951, 37–42.

p. 87 *Invited to lecture at* . . . : William LaJoie, interview with author, 13 April 1994.

p. 87 *Kenny, never a diplomat,* . . . : Albert Deutsch, "The Truth about Sister Kenny," *American Mercury* 59 (November 1944), 610–16.

p. 87 *She also resisted* . . . : Ibid., 611.

p. 87 *"Although the National Foundation . . . "*: Paul, *History of Poliomyelitis*, 343.

p. 88 *A personal conflict between . . .* : Cohn, *Sister Kenny*, 173.

p. 88 *Kenny was called arbitrary, . . .* : Deutsch, "The Truth," 613.

p. 88 *No doubt she could have . . .* : Cohn, *Sister Kenny*, 173.

p. 89 *On the day he should have been . . .* : Keith Dixon, unpublished memoir, "Collected Memories (The Hospital Years)," 1992.

p. 89 *sometimes with the whole process repeated . . .* : "Pain of Polio Relieved," *Science News Letter* 46 (2 September 1944): 146.

p. 89 *Gertrud Svensson Stockton, a physical therapist, . . .* : Gertrud Svensson Stockton, letter to author, [undated] February 1994.

p. 89 *"At times it often seemed to be . . . "*: Jane Stevens, letter to author, 8 February 1994.

p. 90 *Then doctors determined that . . .* : Harry F. Dowling, *Fighting Infection: Conquests of the Twentieth Century* (Cambridge: Harvard University Press, 1977), 207.

p. 90 *most medical people agreed with the NFIP's . . .* : Deutsch, "The Truth," 615.

p. 90 *polio treatment settled into a regimen . . .* : Paul, *History of Poliomyelitis*, 343–44.

p. 90 *followed as soon as possible by exercise . . .* : Dowling, *Fighting Infection*, 207.

p. 91 *Doris Seligman found other particular discomforts . . . .* : Doris Seligman, letter to author, 7 May 1994.

p. 92 *Calling him "the world's most . . . "*: Harold A. Littledale, "Hope and Courage—That Is Warm Springs," *New York Times Sunday Magazine*, (23 January 1944), 9, 30.

p. 92 *"Take the case of a concert pianist . . . "*: Ibid., 30.

p. 93 *Treatment followed one of three . . .* : Davis, *Passage through Crisis*, 50.

p. 94 *The typical physiotherapy plan . . . .* : Following description drawn from Davis, *Passage through Crisis* and "Definitions of Time and Recovery in Paralytic Polio," *American Journal of Sociology LXI* (May 1956): 582–87.

p. 94 *The* Saturday Evening Post *in 1949 ran . . .* : Spencer, "Where Are We Now on Polio?," *Saturday Evening Post*, 17 September 1949, 26.

p. 95 *In many, many cases the gains . . .* : Davis, *Passage through Crisis*, 72.

p. 95 *Dean Williamson, a young* . . . : Dean Williamson, in *Experiments in Survival*, ed. and comp. Edith Henrich (New York: Association for the Aid of Crippled Children, 1961), 24.

p. 95 *Being fitted for braces* . . . : Davis, *Passage through Crisis*, 72.

p. 95 *One boy, an eleven-year-old who* . . . : H. A. Robinson, J. E. Finesinger, and J. S. Bierman, "Psychiatric Considerations in the Adjustment of Patients with Poliomyelitis," *New England Journal of Medicine* 254, no. 21 (1956): 975.

p. 95 *Mary Bready was first fitted* . . . : Mary Bready, unpublished memoirs.

p. 96 *The writer Leonard Kriegel, who contracted* . . . : Leonard Kriegel, *Falling into Life: Essays* (San Francisco: North Point Press, 1991), 8–9.

p. 97 *Just before her polio attack* . . . : Bready, unpublished memoirs.

p. 98 *The American Orthopaedic Association* . . . : Davis, *Passage through Crisis*, 100.

p. 98 *Although many orthopedists privately* . . . : Ibid., footnote 72.

p. 98 *For their part, physiotherapists* . . . : Ibid., 101.

p. 99 *In 1941, for instance, a physician* . . . : "Poliomyelitis: Infantile Paralysis Victims Helped by New Operation," *Scientific American* 164 (April 1941): 202.

p. 99 *Another group of doctors obtained* . . . : "Nerve-Crushing Operation Tried for Chronic Polio," *Science News Letter* 46 (16 September 1944): 187.

p. 100 *Children learned, after being on a ward* . . . : Davis, *Passage through Crisis*, 76.

p. 100 *"The medical costs average* . . . ": Spencer, "Where Are We Now?," 27.

p. 101 *The local chapter in King County,* . . . : *Seattle Times*, 17 January 1954, n.p.

p. 101 *In 1954 the total was over* . . . : *Seattle Times*, 30 January 1955, Section 6, p. 1.

p. 101 *The annual costs for one polio patient* . . . : "Strange Facts about Polio," NFIP. Material appeared in the *Daily Camera*, Boulder, Colorado, 31 January 1956, n.p.

p. 101 *This was at a time when* . . . : David Halberstam, *The Fifties* (New York: Villard Books, 1993), 135.

p. 101 *In 1954 the NFIP gave aid* . . . : Victor Cohn, *Four Billion Dimes*, (Minneapolis, Minn.: Minneapolis Star and Tribune, 1955), 133.

p. 102 *The money was dispensed through* . . . : Ibid., 61.

p. 102 *"It took quite a bit of convincing . . . "*: Thurber, letter to author.

p. 102 *An Arizona boy from the tiny town . . .* : *Arizona Republic*, 16 July 1954, 2.

p. 102 *In one week in 1949 . . .* : "When Polio Strikes," *Newsweek*, 15 August 1949, 6.

p. 104 *The "intense desire to get rid of polio" . . .* : Merle Ross, interview with author.

p. 108 *This out-of-season drive, . . .* : "Money and Polio," *Time*, 23 August 1954, 58.

p. 109 *Some physicians, according to Fred Davis, . . .* : Davis, *Passage through Crisis*, 39.

CHAPTER FIVE: LIFE IMMOBILE

p. 117 *"If we have to wait until the patient . . . "*: "Concentrated Care Fights Polio," *Seattle Times*, 7 January 1954, n.p.

p. 118 *Developed in 1947 . . .* : "Rocking Bed Used for Polio," *Science News Letter* 52 (27 September 1947): 204. Rocking-bed information also from interviews with Marcelle Dunning, August 13 and 14, 1994, and October 5, 1994.

p. 118 *One such stroy was told . . .* : Gene Roehling, as told to Jim Stranger, "I Live in an Iron Lung," *Saturday Evening Post*, 24 March 1951, 138.

p. 120 *"When I laugh I do so . . . "*: Arnold R. Beisser, *Flying without Wings: Personal Reflections on Being Disabled* (New York: Doubleday, 1989), 157.

p. 122 *"Why did my father not . . . "*: Charles L. Mee, *A Visit to Haldeman and Other States of Mind* (New York: M. Evans, 1977), 150.

p. 123 *Baltimore was home to the first one, . . .* : Alice Lake, "They're Learning to Breathe Again," *Saturday Evening Post*, 28 June 1952, 86.

p. 124 *A writer for the* Saturday Evening Post *. . .* : Ibid., 89.

p. 127 *A study done at the Mary MacArthur Respirator Unit . . .* : Dane G. Prugh and Consuelo K. Tagiuri, "Emotional Aspects of the Respirator Care of Patients with Poliomyelitis: Preliminary Report," *Psychosomatic Medicine* 16 (1954): 124.

p. 127 *Norma Duchin, writing about her hospitalization . . .* : Norma Duchin, in Edith Henrich, comp. and ed., *Experiments in Survival* (New York: Association for the Aid of Crippled Children, 1991), 15.

p. 128 *"Physical activity was for them . . . "*: Marcelle Dunning, unpublished paper.

p. 131 *"an extremely painful procedure . . . "*: Beisser, *Flying without Wings*, 53.

p. 134 *The technique, discovered by patients . . .* : "Mental Crippling of Polio," *Science News Letter* 62 (30 August 1952): 132.

p. 134 *In its first year, twenty-two patients, . . .* : Undated, unidentified clipping from Seattle newspaper, from Willa Dee Troester Thoen file.

p. 140 *Lou Sternburg told in his book . . .* : Louis Sternburg, Dorothy Sternburg, and Monica Dickens, *View from the Seesaw* (New York: Dodd, Mead, 1986), 37.

p. 140 *"I had fantasies," he wrote, . . .* : Beisser, *Flying without Wings*, 20.

p. 141 *"I had recurrent fantasies . . . "*: Ibid., 97.

p. 143 *Lou Sternburg's first outing, . . .* : Sternburg, *View from the Seesaw*, 66.

p. 144 *Fears traveled through the rooms, . . .* : Prugh and Tagiuri, "Emotional Aspects," 119.

p. 144 *Researchers at the Mary MacArthur Respirator Unit . . .* : Ibid., 119.

p. 144 *Hospitalized in Baltimore . . .* : Duchin, in Henrich, *Experiments in Survival*, 16.

p. 145 *The NFIP's Morton Seidenfeld, . . .* : Morton A. Seidenfeld, "Psychological Implications of Breathing Difficulties in Poliomyelitis," *American Journal of Orthopsychiatry* 25 (1955): 791–92.

p. 145 *For a few, however, the blood pressure . . .* : B. G. Ferris Jr., P. A. M. Auld, L. Cronkite, H. J. Kaufmann, R. B. Kearsley, M. Prizer, L. Weinstein, "Life Threatening Poliomyelitis," *The New England Journal of Medicine*, 262 (25 February 1960): 372.

p. 145 *For polio patients, however, something . . .* : Marcelle Dunning, interview with author, August 12 and 13, 1994.

p. 146 *Lou Sternburg once had to . . .* : Sternburg, *View from the Seesaw*, 50.

CHAPTER SIX: WEATHERING REALITY

p. 153 *"While the consequences of polio . . . "*: Leonard Kriegel, *Falling into Life: Essays* (San Francisco: North Point Press, 1991), 42.

p. 153 *In my search for what those . . .* : Thanks to Daniel Wilson's essay for directing me to Brody's useful book.

p. 153 *"We are, in an important sense, . . . "*: Howard Brody, *Stories of Sickness*, 182.

p. 154 *She and her husband had the same, . . .* : Mary Bready, unpublished memoir.

p. 155 *Children, even those who came . . .* : Kathleen Allen, "The Responsibility of the Medical Worker to the Poliomyelitis Patient," *Nervous Child* 11, no. 2 (1956): 61.

p. 155 *Even patients who made complete recoveries . . .* : Edith Meyer, "Psychological Considerations in a Group of Children with Poliomyelitis," *Journal of Pediatrics* 31 (1947): 47.

p. 155 *During the first weeks following discharge, . . .* : Ibid., 36.

p. 155 *Children who required prolonged . . .* : Ibid., 47–48.

p. 155 *Mary, the youngest child, and only girl, . . .* : J. Carlton Babbs, letter, 17 October 1952.

p. 156 *one possible "story of sickness" . . . "* Brody, *Stories of Sickness*, 81–85.

p. 157 *Another story of sickness . . .* : Ibid., 83–84.

p. 157 *"In extreme cases . . . "*: Ibid., 84.

p. 158 *"Until I met up with my virus . . . "*: Kriegel, *Falling into Life*, 42–43.

p. 158 *"By the age of nineteen, . . . "*: Ibid., 57.

p. 159 *That year, New York City, . . .* : Naomi Rogers, *Dirt and Disease: Polio before FDR* (New Brunswick, N.J.: Rutgers University Press, 1992), 11.

p. 160 *By the forties it was known . . .* : "Pain of Polio Relieved," *Science News Letter*, 46 (2 September 1944): 146.

p. 160 *In 1949 attendees at a national conference . . .* : "Polio Isolation Period of Only One Week Urged," *Science News Letter* 56 (20 August 1949): 120.

p. 160 *And yet quarantines went on . . .* : Allen, "Responsibility of the Medical Worker," 61.

p. 160 *The actor Mia Farrow . . .* : Ingrid Sischy, "Mia Farrow Has Been Many Things to Many People," *Interview*, April 1994, 81.

p. 161 *"Mad or sane, . . . "*: Kriegel, *Falling into Life*, 183.

p. 162 *As Kriegel pointed out, the views* . . . : Ibid., 184.

p. 162 *For the survivor,* . . . : Ibid.

p. 162 *And yet, he continued, this* . . . : Ibid., 190.

p. 162 *"It is as if the patient thinks* . . . *"*: H. A. Robinson, J. E. Finesinger, and J. S. Bierman, "Psychiatric Considerations in the Adjustment of Patients with Poliomyelitis," *New England Journal of Medicine* 254, no. 21 (1956): 978.

p. 162 *Children in that study* . . . : Ibid.

p. 163 *Polio raced through the rural area* . . . : Jerry Davidoff, "Orange Unaffected by Polio Epidemic," *Tar Heel,* 18 July 1944, 1.

p. 163 *Faced with a growing population* . . . : Carol Hughes, "The Miracle of Hickory," *Coronet,* February 1945, 3–7.

p. 164 *In the summer before his senior year* . . . : Dennis Samson, letter to author, [undated] December 1993.

p. 164 *That was the case at the University of Michigan* . . . : Ruth Hazen, letter to author, 16 April 1994.

p. 165 *Lynda D. W. Bogel recalled* . . . : Lynda D. W. Bogel, letter to author, 12 December 1993.

p. 165 *"raised delicate and precarious issues."*: Fred Davis, *Passage through Crisis: Polio Victims and Their Families* (Indianapolis: Bobbs-Merrill, 1963), 117.

p. 165 *one mother who told Davis* . . . : Ibid., 118.

p. 166 *Davis tells of one mother who* . . . : Ibid., 92.

p. 166 *He tells of another mother* . . . : Ibid., 91.

p. 166 *Such incidents as these* . . . : Ibid., 9.

p. 166 *In an essay based on a study* . . . : Daniel J. Wilson, "Covenants of Work and Grace: Themes of Recovery and Redemption in Polio Narratives," *Literature and Medicine* 13 (Spring 1994): 29.

p. 166 *"the quintessence of the Protestant ideology* . . . *"*: Fred Davis, "Definition of Time and Recovery in Paralytic Polio," *American Journal of Sociology* (1956): 587.

p. 166 *"The gradient structuring of* . . . *"*: Davis, *Passage through Crisis,* 72.

p. 167 *"because they feared that if* . . . *"*: Ibid., 77.

p. 167 *Writing about her friend* . . . : Eleanor Chappell, *On the Shoulders of Giants: The Ben Wright Story* (Philadelphia: Chilton Company, 1960), 23.

p. 167 *One woman I talked to* . . . : Whitney Wing Oppersdorf, letter to author, 18 January 1994.

p. 167 *proved its later undoing*: Davis, *Passage through Crisis*, 104.

p. 168 *"a thief's primer* . . . *"*: Kriegel, *Falling into Life*, 7.

p. 168 *Roosevelt spent the first seven years* . . . : Hugh Gregory Gallagher, *FDR's Splendid Deception* (New York: Dodd, Mead, 1985), 20.

p. 168 *He tried massage,* . . . : Ibid., 24.

p. 168 *Despite all that effort, time, and* . . . : Ibid., 164.

p. 168 *"cavernous room filled with barbells* . . . *"*: Kriegel, *Falling into Life*, 9.

p. 169 *He did hundreds of pushups* . . . : Ibid., 57.

p. 169 *Dorothy Pallas was seven* . . . : Dorothy Pallas, in Edith Henrich, comp. and ed., *Experiments in Survival* (New York: Association for the Aid of Crippled Children, 1991), 88.

p. 169 *illness "is a form of* . . . *"*: Brody, *Stories of Sickness*, 73.

p. 170 *In Daniel Wilson's examination* . . . : Wilson, "Covenants of Work," 25.

p. 171 *Wilson noted that "the failure* . . . *"*: Ibid., 31.

p. 171 *"My breathing was labored,"* . . . : Regina Woods, *Tales from the Iron Lung: And How I Got Out of It* (Philadelphia: University of Pennsylvania Press, 1994), 5.

p. 171 *One, done in 1952* . . . : Dane G. Prugh and Consuelo K. Tagiuri, "Emotional Aspects of the Respirator Care of Patients with Poliomyelitis: Preliminary Report," *Psychosomatic Medicine* 16 (1954): 114.

p. 171 *Patients went through three* . . . : Ibid.

p. 171 *"Nurses and attendants* . . . *"*: Arnold R. Beisser, *Flying without Wings: Personal Reflections on Being Disabled* (New York: Doubleday, 1989), 22.

p. 172 *Marcelle Dunning said she thought* . . . : Dunning, personal correspondence, 26 June 1995.

p. 172 *"the attitudes of families and of the staff* . . . *"*: Prugh and Tagiuri, "Emotional Aspects," 115.

p. 173 *"My whole comfort depends . . . "*: Gene Roehling as told to Jim Stranger, "I Live in an Iron Lung" *Saturday Evening Post*, March 24, 1951, 138.

p. 173 *Arnold Beisser wrote of the . . .* : Beisser, *Flying without Wings*, 18–19.

p. 173 *"like an undeserving outsider . . . "*: Ibid., 37.

p. 174 *"restored to the human community"*: Ibid.

p. 174 *One physician, for example, . . .* : Ibid., 38.

p. 174 *In the polio narratives he studied . . .* : Wilson, "Covenants of Work," 22–41.

p. 174 *"some point in every case . . . "*: Ibid., 23.

p. 174 *Just as the Puritans believed . . .* : Ibid., 24.

p. 174 *the process was "a protracted . . . "*: Ibid., 38.

p. 175 *By observing patients' progress . . .* : Fred Davis, *Passage through Crisis, 49.*

p. 175 *In his study, the probable progress . . .* : Ibid., 84.

p. 175 *Many hospitals deliberately . . .* : Ibid., 64.

p. 176 *One doctor in Davis's study . . .* : Ibid., 84.

p. 176 *A period of about fifteen months . . .* : Ibid., 107.

p. 177 *For some, the fact that they had . . .* : Ibid., 90.

p. 177 *FDR, many years after . . .* : Gallagher, *FDR's Splendid Deception, 69.*

p. 177 *" in our culture it is also an important . . . "*: Davis, *Passage through Crisis*, 64.

p. 177 *One seven-year-old boy . . .* : Ibid., 141–42.

p. 177 *One day Lou Sternburg . . .* : Louis Sternburg, Dorothy Sternburg, and Monica Dickens, *View from the Seesaw* (New York: Dodd, Mead, 1986), 59.

p. 178 *"I suppose we might have been told . . . "*: Kriegel, *Falling into Life*, 6.

p. 178 *Someone took him for an outing . . .* : Sternburg, *View from the Seesaw*, 67.

p. 179 *H. C. A. Lassen, the chief physician . . .* : R. Debre, et al., *Poliomyelitis*, World Health, 1955. Monograph 26, 198.

p. 179 *"Obviously I don't like living . . . "*: Roehling, "I Live in an Iron Lung," 142.

p. 181 *"It's a cliché . . . "*: Jack Clements, letter to author, 9 June 1994.

p. 181 *A social taboo that forbade . . .* : Wilson, "Covenants of Work," 25–26.

p. 181 *In one of the stories for popular magazines . . .* : Ken Purdy, " . . . The Rest of Me Is Alive," *McCall's*, October 1953, 94.

p. 181 *The concept, as outlined by . . .* : Brody, *Stories of Sickness*, 133.

p. 182 *Although the disabled people . . .* : Wilson, "Covenants of Work," 40 n.13.

p. 182 *Roosevelt himself suffered . . .* : Gallagher, *FDR's Splendid Deception*, 22–23.

p. 182 *One of my correspondents, . . .* : Betty Hurwich Zoss, letters to author, 19 December 1993 and 27 January 1994.

p. 182 *Writing to a friend, . . .* : Ken W. Purdy, letter, 7 November 1952.

p. 183 *Families were to play their roles, . . .* : Davis, *Passage through Crisis*, 115–16.

p. 184 *In one recent study, researchers found that . . .* : John G. Bruhn, "Effects of Chronic Illness on the Family," *Journal of Family Practice* 4 (June 1977): 1059.

p. 184 *Families with an ill or handicapped member, . . .* : Brody, *Stories of Sickness*, 111–12.

CHAPTER SEVEN: FORGETTING AND REMEMBERING

p. 194 *Lou Sternburg had a buzzer rigged . . .* : Louis Sternburg, Dorothy Sternburg, and Monica Dickens, *View from the Seesaw*, (New York: Dodd, Mead, 1986), 75, 86.

p. 197 *In their study of respiratory patients, . . .* : Dane G. Prugh and Consuelo K. Tagiuri, "Emotional Aspects of the Respirator Care of Patients with Poliomyelitis: Preliminary Report," *Psychosomatic Medicine* 16 (1954): 114.

p. 198 *"To the severely handicapped, existence itself . . . "*: Pallas, in Edith Henrich, comp. and ed., *Experiments in Survival* (New York: Association for the Aid of Crippled Children, 1991), 89–90.

p. 199 *"Normally endowed people claim . . . "*: Doris Lorenzen, in ibid., 62.

p. 201 *When she brought him home, . . .* : Mary Leonard, interview with author, 18 June 1994.

p. 205 *Of her husband's return home, . . .* : Sternburg, *View from the Seesaw*, 84.

p. 206 *According to Eric Cassell, . . .* : Eric J. Cassell, *The Nature of Suffering: And the Goals of Medicine* (New York: Oxford University Press, 1991), 54.

p. 206 *"the ineluctable forces . . . "*: Ibid.

p. 206 *She could breathe a bit on her own, . . .* : Ted Delaney, "Lily Manning: The Story of a Survivor," *Catholic Digest*, July 1993, 11.

p. 207 *One man, an engineer, . . .* : Elliot Marple, *His Body Broken, His Spirit Afire*, unpublished biography of Alfred Bate Jepson, Bellevue, Washington, April 1992, 5.

p. 208 *"We all recognize certain injuries . . . "*: Cassell, *Nature of Suffering, 44.*

p. 209 *Lou Sternburg wrote that even after . . .* : Sternburg, *View from the Seesaw*, 88.

p. 209 *"There is no doubt that maintaining . . . "*: Ibid., 210.

CHAPTER EIGHT: ANSWERED PRAYERS

p. 214 *Long before there was . . .* : John R. Paul, *A History of Poliomyelitis* (New Haven, Conn.: Yale University Press, 1971), 318.

p. 214 *In 1931 an epidemic . . .* : Geoffrey Marks and William K. Beatty, *Epidemics: The Story of Mankind's Most Lethal and Elusive Enemies from Ancient Times to the Present* (New York: Charles Scribner, 1976), 234.

p. 214 *After first hunting for a polio . . .* : Paul, *History of Poliomyelitis, 98–100.*

p. 215 *In the early forties it was known that . . .* : Harry F. Dowling, *Fighting Infection: Conquests of the Twentieth Century* (Boston: Harvard University Press, 1977), 212.

p. 215 *In the early fifties, with an NFIP grant, . . .* : "Gamma Globulin for Polio," *Scientific American*, June 1953, 50, 52, 54.

p. 215 *Hammon had, however, shown . . .* : Paul, *History of Poliomyelitis*, 394.

p. 215 *The government had classified . . .* : Jane S. Smith, *Patenting the Sun: Polio and the Salk Vaccine* (New York: Morrow, 1990), 174–75.

p. 216 *Around the country, parents like those of . . .* : Roger Beck, letter to author, 6 March 1994.

p. 216 *In Pitman, New Jersey, four cases . . .* : "Mass Polio Inoculations Given," *Seattle Times*, 20 September 1954, 26.

p. 216 *The* Arizona Republic, *reporting that . . .* : *Arizona Republic*, 25 June 1954, n.p.

p. 216 *A committee of experts from . . .* : "G.G. Failed to Halt Polio," *Science News Letter* 65 (6 March 1954): 148.

p. 217 *"Perhaps some day . . . "*: Howard A. Howe, "Are You Afraid of Polio?" *Harper's*, June 1945, 652.

p. 217 *But it was just the sort of job . . .* : Dowling, *Fighting Infection*, 211.

p. 217 *The task began in 1948 . . .* : Victor Cohn, *Four Billion Dimes* (Minneapolis: Minneapolis Star and Tribune, 1955), 97.

p. 217 *Jonas Salk, a physician who was . . .* : Ibid.

p. 217 *As many as 196 had been suspected . . .* : Dowling, *Fighting Infection*, 211; and Paul, *History of Poliomyelitis*, 234.

p. 217 *The second important piece of the puzzle . . .* : "Studies Averted Damage to Brain," *New York Times*, 13 April 1955, 21.

p. 217 *Since antibodies form in blood, . . .* : Ibid.

p. 217 *Dorothy M. Horstmann at Yale . . .* : Dowling, *Fighting Infection*, 211.

p. 218 *By 1952, Salk had been satisfied . . .* : Cohn, *Four Billion Dimes*, 101.

p. 218 *Injecting children, among them his own, . . .* : "Shy, Quiet, Confident Dr. Salk Often Worked 18 Hours a Day," *New York Times*, 13 April 1955, 21.

p. 218 *They had poured an average of . . .* : Dowling, *Fighting Infection*, 214.

p. 219 *Between 1938 and 1955 . . .* : "Roosevelt Established a Vast Foundation, Unit Has Grown to 3,100 Chapters," *New York Times*, 13 April 1955, 24.

p. 220 *March passed. Then on April . . .* : Smith, *Patenting the Sun*, 256–57; and Cohn, *Four Billion Dimes*, 122.

p. 221 *"To those who were making the decision, . . . "*: Smith, *Patenting the Sun*, 258.

p. 221 *"In all the literature that surrounded . . . "*: Ibid., 22.

p. 221 *Thousands of little vials* . . . : Cohn, *Four Billion Dimes*, 124.

p. 222 *First, some were given blood tests* . . . : "O Pioneers!" *New Yorker* 30 (8 May 1954): 24–25.

p. 223 *"No top secret during the war* . . . *"*: "Finding Due Today on Polio Vaccine," *New York Times*, 12 April 1955, 1.

p. 223 *"a short, chunky man* . . . *"*: "Fanfare Ushers Verdict on Tests," *New York Times*, 13 April 1955, 1.

p. 223 *Although he spoke in a* . . . : Ibid., 20.

p. 224 *"It's a great day.* . . . *"*: "6 Vaccine Makers Get U.S. Licenses," *New York Times*, 13 April 1955, 1.

p. 224 *An official from the American* . . . : "Leaders of A.M.A. Hail Vaccine Test," *New York Times*, 13 April 1955, 20.

p. 224 *Eleanor Roosevelt placed a wreath* . . . : "Mrs. Roosevelt Pleased by Salk Test Outcome," *New York Times*, 13 April 1955, 20.

p. 224 *Word that the Salk vaccine* . . . : "It Came Too Late for Them," *Seattle Post-Intelligencer*, 13 April 1955, 1.

p. 225 *"The development of polio vaccines,* . . . *"*: Cohn, *Four Billion Dimes*, 7.

p. 225 *An editorial in the* New York Times . . . : "Dawn of a New Medical Day," *New York Times*, 13 April 1955, 28.

p. 226 *"The vaccine will be scarcer* . . . *"*: "Seattle Children Get Salk-Vaccine Shots," *Seattle Times*, 13 April 1955, 1.

p. 226 *"Psychology Gives Way to Nickel* . . . *"*: *Seattle Times*, late April, 1955.

p. 227 *Cutter Laboratories announced a special* . . . : Smith, *Patenting the Sun*, 362.

p. 228 *some four-hundred thousand polio inoculations* . . . : Paul, *History of Poliomyelitis*, 435.

p. 228 *Nonetheless, what seemed unthinkable* . . . : Paul, 437.

p. 228 *She had been inoculated* . . . : Frank Lynch, "The Miracle of Modern Medicine That Failed for Little Girl," *Seattle Post-Intelligencer*, 22 August 1955, 17.

p. 229 *That some live virus might* . . . : Smith, *Patenting the Sun*, 359–64.

p. 229 *The responses to the Cutter incident* . . . : Ibid., 360–61.

p. 229 *Some of them were inaccurate, . . .* : "Serum Scare Abates," *Daily Camera*, 28 April 1955, 1.

p. 229 *Other people concluded, . . .* : Smith, *Patenting the Sun*, 364.

p. 229 *In one way or another, enough parents . . .* : Paul, *History of Poliomyelitis*, 438.

p. 230 *Karen McGinnis, whose mother . . .* : McGinnis, letter to author.

p. 230 *One woman's physician-husband . . .* : Ted Delaney, "Lily Manning: The Story of a Survivor," *Catholic Digest*, July 1993, 7.

p. 230 *just like Bill Warwick . . .* : James Warwick, letter to author.

p. 230 *The vaccine brought a drastic drop . . .* : "Polio Decline," *Time*, 12 August 1957, 62; and 21 October 1957, 70.

p. 230 *In a decade, the number of annual cases . . .* : Geoffrey Marks and William K. Beatty, *Epidemics: The Story of Mankind's Most Lethal and Elusive Enemies from Ancient Times to the Present* (New York: Charles Scribner, 1976), 236.

p. 231 *On the same day that newspapers . . .* : "Foundation to Go On," *New York Times*, April 13, 1955, 24.

p. 231 *The drive toward nationwide immunization . . .* : Smith, *Patenting the Sun*, 364.

p. 231 *That year, sixty-seven million . . .* : "Polio Decline," *Time*, 21 October 1957, 70.

p. 231 *In the fall of 1957 . . .* : "Doctors to Mail Polio Reminder Cards in Color," *Science News Letter* 72 (November 1957): 313.

p. 232 *Elvis Presley agreed to be vaccinated . . .* : Smith, *Patenting the Sun*, 371.

p. 232 *HEW Secretary Marion B. Folsom . . .* : "Polio Decline," *Time*, 21 October 1957, 70.

p. 232 *"I am compelled to add my personal plea . . . "*: Frances Downing Vaughan, clipping sent to author.

p. 232 *By the spring of 1958, as the polio season . . .* : "Polio-Dangerous Lag," *Newsweek* 5 May 1958, 70.

p. 232 *In August that year $25 million . . .* : "Polio and Apathy," *Newsweek*, 25 August 1958, 52.

p. 232 *Almost five hundred cases of polio, . . .* : "Why the Polio Outbreak," *Newsweek*, 6 October 1958, 52–53.

p. 233 *In the meantime, the nation was getting . . .* : The history of the live virus vaccine, except where noted, is drawn from Paul, *History of Poliomyelitis*, 441–56.

p. 233 *Sabin reported in 1957 . . .* : "Need Live Virus Vaccine to Stop Spread of Polio," *Science News Letter* 72 (July 1957): 40.

p. 233 *The refusal of the NFIP . . .* : Paul, *History of Poliomyelitis*, 345.

p. 233 *By 1962 the Sabin vaccine . . .* : Dowling, *Fighting Infection*, 218; and Paul, *History of Poliomyelitis*, 466.

p. 234 *While Salk's contribution had been . . .* : Smith, *Patenting the Sun*, 149.

p. 234 *One in four million doses . . .* : Ibid., 386.

p. 234 *When the Sabin-type vaccine . . .* : Paul, *History of Poliomyelitis*, 466.

p. 234 *The recommendation from the advisory committee . . .* : Ibid., 467.

p. 234 *Salk was criticized, called . . .* : Cohn, *Four Billion Dimes*, 106.

p. 234 *"It left a slightly bitter taste . . . "*: Dowling, *Fighting Infection*, 219.

p. 235 *It is a controversy over the issues . . .* : Naomi Rogers, *Dirt and Disease: Polio before FDR* (New Brunswick, N.J.: Rutgers University Press, 1992), 186.

p. 235 *But because it never enters the intestines, . . .* : Daniel Jack Chasan, "The Polio Paradox," *Science 86*, April 1986, 37.

p. 235 *The picture is not complete, however, . . .* : Ibid.

p. 236 *"at a time when omens were . . . "*: Paul, *History of Poliomyelitis*, 318.

p. 236 *Hundreds of iron lungs, . . .* : Stanley M. Vlanoff, *MATS: The Story of the Military Air Transport Service* (New York: Franklin Watts, 1964), 114–15.

p. 236 *"Somehow, polio had ceased . . . "*: Smith, *Patenting the Sun*, 371.

CHAPTER NINE: SILENCES

p. 243 *"You can heave your spirit . . . "*: Annie Dillard, *Pilgrim at Tinker Creek* (New York: HarperPerennial, 1985), 3.

p. 245 *"Suddenly," he told me, . . .* : Clements, letter to author, 9 June 1994.

p. 246 *One such patient was Al Jepson.*: Unpublished biography of Al Jepson.

p. 247 *the anniversary reaction*: David P. Phillips, Camilla A. Van Voorhees, and Todd E. Ruth, "The Birthday: Lifeline or Deadline?" *Psychosomatic Medicine* 54 (1992): 532–42.

p. 247 *"we rarely go gentle . . . "*: Sherwin B. Nuland, *How We Die: Reflections on Life's Final Chapter* (New York: Knopf, 1994), 9.

p. 247 *Even when someone yearns . . .* : Ibid., 233–34.

p. 248 *In their study of respirator patients . . .* : Dane G. Prugh and Consuelo K. Tagiuri, "Emotional Aspects of the Respirator Care of Patients with Poliomyelitis: Preliminary Report," *Psychosomatic Medicine* 16 (1954): 114.

p. 248 *"If the suffering was severe . . . "*: Eric J. Cassell, *The Nature of Suffering: And the Goals of Medicine* (New York: Oxford University Press, 1991), 54.

p. 253 *The French writer Albert Camus . . .* : quoted in Nuland, *How We Die*, 200.

p. 254 *In his memoir, . . .* : Wilfrid Sheed, *In Love with Daylight: A Memoir of Recovery* (New York: Simon & Schuster, 1995), 36–37.

CHAPTER TEN: AFTERMATH

p. 256 *Some 250,000 people . . .* : Marinos C. Dalakas, Harry Bartfeld, and Leonard T. Kurland, "Polio Redux," *The Sciences*, July/August 1995, 32.

p. 256 *As for the 1.4 million . . .* : Ibid., 32.

p. 256 *The world has seen . . .* : N. Ward, J. Milstien, H. Hull, B. Hull, "A Global Overview and Hope for the Eradication of Poliomyelitis by the Year 2000," *Tropical and Geographical Medicine* 45, no. 5 (1993): 200–201.

p. 256 *These days, all cases in the United States . . .* : W. H. Foege, "A World without Polio," *Journal of the American Medical Association* 270, no. 15, (1993): 1859–60.

p. 256 *The last known case in all the Americas . . .* : "Americas declared a polio-free zone," *New Scientist*, 8 October 1994, 4.

p. 256 *In addition to the Americas, other areas . . .* : Ward et al., "Global Overview," 201.

p. 257 *A high percentage . . .* : Ibid.

p. 257 *Among world health authorities,* . . . : William H. Foege, "A World without Polio," *Journal of the American Medical Association* 270, no. 15 (20 October 1993): 1859–60.

p. 257 *The methods to stop it* . . . : Ward et al., "Global Overview," 201.

p. 257 *Although smallpox is the only* . . . : Peter R. Wright, Robert J. Kim-Farley, Ciro A. de Quadros, Susan E. Robertson, Robert McN. Scott, Nicholas A. Ward, and Ralph H. Henderson, "Strategies for the Global Eradication of Poliomyelitis by the Year 2000," *New England Journal of Medicine* 325 (19 December 1991): 1779.

p. 257 *But polio is different* . . . : Melissa Hendricks, "The Wizard of Public Health," *Johns Hopkins Magazine*, February 1991, 15–23.

p. 257 *The oral polio vaccine,* . . . : Wright et al., "Global Eradication," 1774, 1778.

p. 257 *In the 1950s, polio had* . . . : Fred Davis, *Passage through Crisis: Polio Victims and Their Families* (Indianapolis: Bobbs-Merrill, 1963), 4-5.

p. 258 *"There has never been a disease* . . . *"*: Sherwin B. Nuland, *How We Die: Reflections on Life's Final Chapter* (New York: Knopf, 1994), 172.

p. 258 *The cost of treating even a fraction* . . . : Ward et al., "Global Overview," 198.

p. 258 *And by the turn of the century,* . . . : Peter Jareb, "Viruses: On the Edge of Life, on the Edge of Death," *National Geographic*, July 1994, 85.

p. 258 *Even now, more than a decade later,* . . . : Dalakas et al., "Polio Redux," 33.

p. 259 *Although nothing was said of it at the time,* . . . : Hugh Gregory Gallagher, *FDR's Splendid Deception* (New York: Dodd, Mead, 1985), 189.

p. 259 *What causes the syndrome is not clear* . . . : Eric J. Cassell, *The Nature of Suffering: And the Goals of Medicine* (New York: Oxford University Press, 1991), 49.

p. 260 *Although one study showed* . . . : Mohammad K. Sharief, Romain Hentges, and Maria Ciardi, "Intrathecal Immune Response in Patients with the Post-Polio Syndrome," *New England Journal of Medicine* 325 (12 September 1991): 749–55.

p. 260 *"The very toughness on which* . . . *"*: Jane S. Smith, *Patenting the Sun: Polio and the Salk Vaccine* (New York: Morrow, 1990), 383.

p. 260 *No one has studied the issue, but based* . . . : Dalakas et al., "Polio Redux," 34.

p. 260 *why, even, it was a summertime* . . . : Foege, "World without Polio," 1859–60.

p. 261 *A writer for* . . . : Philip Elmer-Dewitt, "Reliving Polio," *Time*, 28 March 1994, 54.

p. 261 *"Many of us never got* . . . ": Ibid.

p. 261 *"shook his fist at the fates* . . . ": Gallagher, *FDR's Splendid Deception*, 27.

p. 261 *FDR convinced "his family* . . . ": Ibid., 213.

p. 261 *"A visible paralytic handicap* . . . ": Ibid., xi.

p. 261 *When Roosevelt's Hyde Park,* . . . : Ibid., 209.

P. 262 *So thoroughly have we expunged* . . . : David Halberstam, *The Fifties* (New York: Villard Books, 1993).

p. 262 *In his study of polio narratives,* . . . : Daniel H. Wilson, "Covenants of Work and Grace: Themes of Recovery and Redemption in Polio Narratives," *Literature and Medicine* 13, no. 1 (1994), 38.

SELECTED
BIBLIOGRAPHY

Beisser, Arnold R. *Flying without Wings: Personal Reflections on Being Disabled*. New York: Doubleday, 1989.

Brody, Howard, M.D. *Stories of Sickness*. New Haven, Conn.: Yale University Press, 1987.

Cassell, Eric J. *The Nature of Suffering: And the Goals of Medicine*. New York: Oxford University Press, 1991.

Cohn, Victor. *Four Billion Dimes*. Minneapolis: Minneapolis Star and Tribune, 1955.

Cohn, Victor. *Sister Kenny: The Woman Who Challenged the Doctors*. Minneapolis: University of Minnesota Press, 1975.

Davis, Fred. "Definitions of Time and Recovery in Paralytic Polio." *American Journal of Sociology* (1956): 582–87.

Davis, Fred. *Passage through Crisis: Polio Victims and Their Families*. Indianapolis: Bobbs-Merrill, 1963.

Dowling, Harry F. *Fighting Infection: Conquests of the Twentieth Century*. Cambridge, Mass.: Harvard University Press, 1977.

Gallagher, Hugh Gregory. *FDR's Splendid Deception*. New York: Dodd, Mead, 1985.

Hall, Robert F. *Through the Storm: A Polio Story*. St. Cloud, Minn.: North Star Press, 1990.

Henrich, Edith, comp. and ed. *Experiments in Survival*. New York: Association for the Aid of Crippled Children, 1991.

Howe, Howard A. "Are You Afraid of Polio?" *Harper's*, June 1945, 646–53.

Howe, Howard A. "Can We Vaccinate against Polio?" *Harper's*, April 1951, 37–42.

Kriegel, Leonard. *Falling into Life: Essays*. San Francisco: North Point Press, 1991.

Marks, Geoffrey, and William K. Beatty. *Epidemics: The Story of Mankind's Most Lethal and Elusive Enemies from Ancient Times to the Present*. New York: Charles Scribner, 1976.

Nuland, Sherwin B. *How We Die: Reflections on Life's Final Chapter*. New York: Knopf, 1994.

Paul, John R., *A History of Poliomyelitis*. New Haven, Conn.: Yale University Press, 1971.

Prugh, Dane G., and Consuelo K. Tagiuri, "Emotional Aspects of the Respirator Care of Patients with Poliomyelitis: Preliminary Report." *Psychosomatic Medicine* 16 (1954): 104–28.

Purdy, Ken. " ' . . . The Rest of Me Is Alive.' " *McCall's*, October 1953, 32–35, 58, 60, 62, 71, 74, 82, 86, 87, 92, 93.

Purdy, Ken. "What Are Little Boys Made Of?" *Reader's Digest*, March 1953, 42–44.

Robinson, H. A., J. E. Finesinger, and J. S. Bierman. "Psychiatric Considerations in the Adjustment of Patients with Poliomyelitis." *New England Journal of Medicine* 254, no. 21 (1956): 975–80.

Rogers, Naomi. *Dirt and Disease: Polio before FDR*. New Brunswick, N.J.: Rutgers University Press, 1992.

Smith, Jane S. *Patenting the Sun: Polio and the Salk Vaccine*. New York: Morrow, 1990.

Spencer, Steven M. "The Best News Yet on Polio!" *Saturday Evening Post*, 1 November 1952, 25, 129, 131, 132, 134.

Spencer, Steven M. "Where Are We Now on Polio?" *Saturday Evening Post*, 17 September 1949, 26, 27, 87, 89, 90, 91, 93.

Sternburg, Louis, Dorothy Sternburg, and Monica Dickens. *View from the Seesaw*. New York: Dodd, Mead, 1986.

Ward, Geoffrey C. *A First Class Temperament: The Emergence of Franklin Roosevelt*. New York: Harper & Row, 1989.

Ward, N., J. Milstien, H. Hull, B. Hull, "A Global Overview and Hope for the Eradication of Poliomyelitis by the Year 2000." *Tropical and Geographical Medicine* 45, no. 5 (1993): 200–201.

Wilson, Daniel J. "Covenants of Work and Grace: Themes of Recovery and Redemption in Polio Narratives." *Literature and Medicine* 13, no. 1 (1994): 22–41.

INDEX

A

Abandonment, fears of, 198, 250
Acceptance (of illness), 174–75
"Acidify bags," 44
Acute paralytic poliomyelitis
  sequelae, 258
Adaptation (to illness), 174–75
Adelphi Hospital (Brooklyn, NY), 85
Adults, polio and, 27, 126
AIDS, 26, 42, 114, 161, 258
Air travel, iron lung patients, 77–79,
  113–15
Alum, 36, 44
American Medical Association
  (AMA), 32, 224, 231
American Weekly (magazine), 85
Amusement parks. *See* Public
  gathering places
Angell, James Emerson, 129
Angell, Marylin, 129, 143, 144, 207
Ann Arbor (MI), respirator center in,
  123
Anniversary reaction, 247
Anterior horn cells, 16
Arkansas, polio epidemic, 81
Arms, effects of polio on, 16, 43
Armstrong, Charles, 36

B

Babbs, J. Carlton, Harriet, and Mary,
  155, 163
Baldwin, Dorothy, 224

Baldwin, Jeanne, 225
Beck, Roger, 216
Beisser, Arnold
  about, 56
  as iron lung patient, 60, 71–72,
    120
  physical therapy, pain of, 131
  reaction to illness, 140–41, 171,
    173–74
Billings, Frances. *See* Finke,
  Frances Billings
Black, Delbert (Del)
  about, 1–2
  alcohol use, 5, 58, 138, 197
  arrival in Seattle, 121, 122–23
  childhood/school years, 12
  marriage, 6–7, 13, 121–22
  military service, 12–13
  reaction to wife's illness/death,
    134–35, 136–40, 196–98, 248,
    253
Black, Jesse, 12, 137
Black, Ken (Kenny)
  early years, 4–7, 121
  grandparents and, 248–49
  mother's illness/death and, 136,
    138, 141, 186, 189, 192, 208,
    210, 238, 240, 251
  receives polio vaccine, 230
Black, Maud, 12, 138–39, 141
Black, Roland, 138
Black, Virginia Royce
  (Mrs. Delbert)
  acute phase, polio, 7–19